Navigating the C

Navigating the C:

A Nurse Charts the Course for Cancer Survivorship Care

By Alene Nitzky, Ph.D., RN, OCN

Blue Bayou Press

Navigating the C: A Nurse Charts the Course for Cancer Survivorship Care and its contents, including all materials in the Cancer Harbors® and FIERCE: Functional & Fit, Independent, Energized, Restored, Confident, Empowered® programs, videos, printed, online, and downloadable materials, are not medical advice or nursing care. For medical advice, consult a licensed physician.

Although the author and publisher have made every effort to ensure that the information in this book was correct at press time, the author and publisher do not assume and hereby disclaim any liability to any party for any loss, damage, or disruption caused by errors or omissions, whether such errors or omissions result from negligence, accident, or any other cause.

Published by Blue Bayou Press LLC

978-1-943889-08-2 (Paperback)
978-1-943889-09-9 (Kindle)

Credits
Content Advising: Jean Lehmann, Ph.D., and Ken Smith, Ed.D.
Copy Editing: Andrea Morris, AM Writing Consulting
Cover Design: Kevin Heyse, Sage Marketing Group, Inc.

In memory of Cathy Morgan, 1947-2017

Dedication

For my Dad, Sheldon Nitzky, who taught me how to endure, and my husband, Dennis Leck, who breathes perseverance.

Acknowledgements

A book is never written alone. The clients and patients I've worked with since 2001 have my utmost gratitude for their honesty and willingness to share many personal details, sometimes of considerable discomfort and suffering, and often of joy and relief. Thanks to Ken Smith and Jean Lehmann for reviewing the manuscript as it was written, and for their advice and support along the way, Julia Blyumkin and the team at Sage Marketing Group for their wisdom, wizardry, and cover design, and the wonderful team of cancer survivors who reviewed Cancer Harbors as it was originally developed: Megan Dell, MD, Melissa Brown, RN, Nguyen Nguyen, Jane Kinney, Terri Coutee of Diep C Journey, and special thanks to Anna Clauson for her tireless efforts in developing the Cancer Harbors video library.

I also want to thank the members of FIERCE in Fort Collins, Colorado, for their participation and dedication to the program since it began in October 2014, Martin Johns and Bridget Holt of Raintree Athletic Club in Fort Collins for their generosity in providing the space for FIERCE since its inception and sustaining it with their support, and Denise P. for being the catalyst. Thanks to the many community providers and volunteers who donate their time and talents to make FIERCE a unique learning experience. Thanks to Mary Vivo and Leah Barrett at Hope Lives! for providing Cancer Harbors as a service to their clients, to Jeneane Malone, BSN, RN, OCN, and Lisa Bliss, MD, for their insights into the physician and nurse experience in healthcare, and to Rachael Coffren for keeping me focused forward at the right moments, and inward when needed.

I also want to thank Andrew Lopez, RN, and the nurse entrepreneurs at Nurseup.com who have become my colleagues. Special thanks to Amelia J. Roberts, BSN, RN, of Solutions by Amelia for being a social marketing whiz and coming up with a great title for the book, Lisbeth Overton, BSN, RN, and to Kristin Carroll and Jillian Schmitt of Survivorship Solutions for their shared vision and enthusiastic support. I have enormous gratitude for Mark Roby, PA-C, my most ardent critic, for his crucial input at key junctures in the writing of this book. I also want to thank Bonnie Burris, Lisa Falsetto, Vicki Fisbeck, Liz Westers, Brian Miller, RD, and John Garnand, and the members of Sharing the Cancer Journey, and Kirsten Schuster, Dale Perry, Dave Williams, Hayley Weiss-Dubin, Christine Orr, Troy Bryant, and Christopher O'Loughlin, for their support, generosity, and wisdom. Special thanks to my fellow nurses Judy Tooley and Susan Smith for their soothing presence, and to Jan and the late Rick Johnson for their inspiration and validation. Thanks to Apryl Allen for her insights and stories, Carol Bush at Healthcare Marketing Network, my publisher and coach Deanna Cooper Gillingham of Blue Bayou Press for her guidance through the entire process, and Andrea Morris for her patience and care in meticulously editing and formatting the manuscript into something I never could have achieved in a lifetime! Thanks to Barbara Dyer Brown for when I needed time to recharge, and to the many others who have been influential, please know that your insights and support are much appreciated.

Foreword

A cancer diagnosis often forces survivors and co-survivors to acknowledge their primal desire to live...the focus of daily life shifting entirely to treating the disease. Meanwhile, life falls apart.

There are more than 15½ million cancer survivors in the United States today, and that number is growing due to scientific advances in medicine and technology. Many of these survivors are left with significant physical, emotional, and financial impairments related to their cancer and cancer treatments. In addition, co-survivors experience side effects as often, and sometimes more deeply, than the patients they support. These hardships can significantly decrease the quality of life for all involved, yet are often overlooked or marginalized within our healthcare systems.

Providers and oncology teams have not lost sight of the importance of caring for people with cancer. Rather, they face increasing pressure as their responsibilities have shifted to managing multiple priorities with considerably less resources. Cancer is an exceptionally complex disease, compelling patients and caregivers to navigate multiple services, while requiring providers to align teams from numerous departments. Often, healthcare systems lack the implementation of coordinated survivorship services that effectively drive better outcomes as patients recover from side effects related to cancer. As a result, when medical treatment is stabilized or ceased, survivors may feel abandoned and overwhelmed as they attempt to regain their lifestyle and independence.

Written from the vantage point of a passionate, patient-focused oncology nurse, *Navigating the C* affords readers the opportunity to evolve beyond a typical disease-centric viewpoint to one prioritizing overall wellness and quality of life. Dr. Nitzky firmly encourages us to consider the "big picture" of optimal patient care, rather than simply checking off boxes to meet minimal requirements or to support faux appearances and accolades. She states, "Let's venture beyond merely treating disease. We must transcend the survivorship care plan to reduce the risk of recurrence or co-morbid conditions, to help patients enjoy better health and quality of life, and to truly heal patients whose diseases have been treated."

Our company, Survivorship Solutions, was founded on the same principles—that coordinated survivorship services should be prioritized over medical treatments alone. Our experience as physical therapists and long-time providers of high-quality cancer rehabilitation fosters our belief that survival is not simply a "disease-free" state, but that physical, functional, emotional, sexual, financial, and social impairments must also be alleviated, allowing patients to thrive. However, meaningful change cannot happen without both intention and action. The medical community must want to implement strategies that improve the cancer patient experience, and they must seek out the best methods for doing so.

Navigating the C is a valuable resource for patients, caregivers, healthcare professionals, and other oncology stakeholders. Dr. Nitzky offers her respected insights and solutions for implementing change and integrating coordinated interdisciplinary care. She provides a unique perspective as an exercise enthusiast, educator, oncology nurse, and patient herself. Her aim is to ensure that people and their loved ones affected by cancer are prioritized by implementing four "CARE" principles: creativity, authenticity, resourcefulness, and empathy. She addresses many of the pink elephants polluting our cancer centers, such as the high cost of cancer treatments without true consideration of financial strain versus benefit to the patients receiving them. She urges providers to utilize palliative care solutions, which value and maximize quality of life, and to embrace, rather than avoid, uncomfortable discussions relating to end-of-life. She also endorses the need for greater nursing autonomy, since oncology nurses are most often the team members who recommend and reinforce interventions and therapies that result in increased patient advocacy, empowerment, and wellness.

In the world of cancer survivorship, we have come a long way, both medically and as providers of specialty services. National organizations and associations have augmented these efforts by implementing standards that help drive consistent, high-quality cancer care. Many healthcare systems have become better at approaching survivors holistically, viewing them as unique individuals with complex needs to help them control their disease and alleviate unnecessary suffering. Still, too many others continue to overlook essential survivorship care services, allowing people to fall through the cracks of a fragmented system.

Navigating the C is an honest look at where we are now, our vision of ideal survivorship care, and the steps we must take to get there. Hospital administrators, policy makers, patient advocates, healthcare professionals, caregivers, and patients will all benefit from the solutions recommended by Dr. Nitzky to embrace a better way of caring for our patients so that they may achieve their optimal health and potential.

Kristin M. Carroll, PT

Jillian Schmitt, MSPT

Founders of Survivorship Solutions, LLC
An innovative cancer rehabilitation and survivorship services consulting firm

Preface

This book came about from going in circles.

As an ultra-endurance runner, I enjoy the meditative and spiritual nature of long runs. Sometimes I run for days around the same loop. One of my favorite places to run is a local cemetery with a flat, one-mile, unpaved road around the perimeter. It allows me to think, or to not think. Mostly it clears my head; all I must do is move forward. It is great spiritual practice for me, and it sets the stage for my creative pursuits.

At times, I feel like I've lived in two worlds: one is the professional, driven, competitive world that builds status, salaries, resumes, and credentials trailing one's name—the one of healthcare as we know it today. The other is the creative, intangible, and difficult-to-quantify world. These two worlds counter each other: structure versus freedom, rules versus creativity, policy versus spirit, stifling versus expressive, ego-based versus interconnected.

I have been a doctoral student, educator, coach, exercise trainer for people with chronic health conditions, nurse, and business owner. I have also been a writer, artist, and athlete over the same time frame. For the past 15 years, I have experienced the healthcare system in different roles: a tangential observer, a patient, a family member and caregiver of people with cancer, a nursing student, and finally as a nurse in critical care and oncology. I am not, however, a cancer survivor. I have been fortunate to have never had cancer myself, at this point in my life.

The reader might ask, why write this book if you are not a cancer survivor?

The purpose of this book is to present a different approach to thinking about cancer survivorship care. I intend to provoke thought about surviving cancer in our existing healthcare system, to encourage action, and to avoid unnecessary trauma in the event of a cancer diagnosis. I also aim to unite all stakeholders in healthcare to build a system that improves health, quality of life, and outcomes around cancer survivorship, while reducing healthcare costs.

The acronym CARE describes this strategy: If we approach health with creativity, authenticity, resourcefulness, and empathy, at all levels of the healthcare system, we will waste less and get more. To do this, we must examine our values and work together in mutual respect and interdisciplinary collaboration to solve the problems that lead to gaps in cancer survivorship care. Real collaboration allows our voices to be heard equally, with cancer survivors' outcomes foremost in mind.

On a Saturday morning in January, the cemetery is quiet. Expansive, old, leafless trees and long, pyramidal blue spruce and pines stand guard, deserted by birds. This is a place of peace.

As the sun rises, I can see the names on snow-topped headstones. I am reminded of the people buried here whom I knew as patients. I remember them for who they were and the stories their families told me, and often I am surprised at how much detail I remember. Some suffered much more than they should have. Some accepted mortality gracefully. Some refused to let go, leading to tragic and painful, not to mention expensive, ends.

I come full circle around the cemetery one more time, as I have come full circle in my life's work. I hope this book shows the world the value of creativity, authenticity, resourcefulness, and empathy in caring for cancer survivors' needs. That is my mission.

Alene Nitzky
Fort Collins, Colorado
January 25, 2017

Introduction

"Wherever you go, there you are."

– Jon Kabat-Zinn[1]

As an oncology nurse working as a health and support coach for people with cancer, during and after treatment, I answer the basic questions they often ask. Those are:

» What can I do to succeed in getting through my treatment?

» What can I do to reduce the chances of the cancer coming back?

» What can I do to recover my way of life prior to my diagnosis?

» Is there anything I could have done differently?

None of these questions have simple answers, and each individual case is different. But healthcare professionals have done a poor job of addressing people's individual needs for guidance, support, and information on these topics, despite an overabundance of information online and throughout our communities. This book guides and directs you in sorting through that information.

I've spent several years working in the community with people who are healing from the various traumas inflicted by their experiences as cancer patients within the healthcare system. Again and again I hear stories and questions about the fears and struggles of cancer that don't ever seem to be addressed. This book addresses those fears and struggles.

Nearly 40 percent of us will be diagnosed with cancer at some point in our lives. Many of these

---

1   Kabat-Zinn, 2005

people will experience feelings of loss of control, shock, and mental paralysis when they are diagnosed. Let's try to keep these feelings to a minimum. We buy insurance for floods or fires even in places where they rarely happen, but we do not prepare ourselves for cancer even though it affects so many of us personally, and nearly everyone secondarily. This book explains how to prepare for the experience, even before you may need it.

In the appendix, I have included samples of the FIERCE and Cancer Harbors programs I developed. I also propose a basic cancer literacy curriculum, called Prevent-Prepare-Prehab, for people who have never had cancer but wish to build their knowledge and skills around it.

The Cancer Harbors sample modules are presented to demonstrate the contents, whom they serve best, and how they work. I am collecting preliminary data on both programs, in the interest of pursuing research trials to study the impact of these programs on quality of life, outcomes, and healthcare costs. To that end, I have also included a brief discussion of the theoretical underpinnings in the appendix.

This book is written from a nurse's perspective, about how each of the stakeholders in the current healthcare system—nurses, physicians, executives and administrators, cancer patients, and people who have never had cancer—can do a better job of meeting people's needs around cancer.

I do not intend to single out any group of stakeholders to blame for the problems we have. Instead, I share stories of what I have observed to begin a discussion on possible changes and improvements. I offer solutions wherever possible. If we are to have a system that works for us, instead of doing to us and taking from us, we all need to be aware, informed, and vocal.

Nurses' perspectives often get lost in discussions about healthcare, deferring instead to physicians, administrators, and other high-status players in the game. Nurses are the professionals who work most closely with patients, however. We are trained holistically to recognize and relieve suffering. Our first concern is patient safety. We advocate for patients. Nurses are in the eye of the storm, and we rely on both quantitative and qualitative information to provide our care. Without nurses, patients would be adrift at sea. Our voices should be heard.

Our current big business approach to healthcare shortchanges not only current and future patients but also direct care providers who want to help people. The system is creating moral distress among physicians, nurses, and others who provide services. It is important for patients and citizens to see how these constraints impact their care.

This is not a mainstream book. It is not intended to change your mind if you believe that traditional Western approaches to medicine have all the answers, that the current healthcare system's business model approach is working well, that your doctor knows everything needed to provide for your complete well-being and recovery before, during, and after cancer treatment, or that healthcare and medicine are a linear, predictable process that has clearly defined answers.

This book is for you if:

» You believe in science and evidence-based medicine but feel there needs to be a more holistic and timely approach to solving the problems we create through our medical interventions.

» You have ever questioned why communication with your doctor and healthcare providers is difficult or incomplete, even if you feel they have done an excellent job in your treatment.

» Your health concerns have ever been dismissed or discounted, or you failed to follow through or get a referral to get your concerns addressed.

» You are trying to recover your health, energy, and quality of life after cancer treatment but have not found the answers from your doctor.

» You fear cancer but would like to know more about it so you can reduce the risk for yourself and your family, or support someone else who has cancer.

» You have no idea how you would handle a serious illness diagnosis for yourself or a family member, as a patient or a caregiver.

» You wish you knew what questions to ask your doctor, or how to find good health information, products, and services.

» You feel that the lengthy process of building bodies of evidence to influence changes in practice is not adequately serving the needs of those suffering from cancer now.

» You are a community provider of support services or health and wellness services and would like to know more about the healthcare system's approach to cancer to better support cancer survivors.

» You are a healthcare provider (physician, nurse, social worker, mental health worker, or other professional) and you feel that the current system is shortchanging you and your patients and would like ideas for improvement.

My goals for this book are:

1. For everyone to define their own values around health, life, healthcare, and mortality, so they can be clear about what they want and need to do in the unfortunate event of a cancer diagnosis, by asking the following questions:

   - How do I define "health"?
   - What does it mean to be healthy?
   - What are the benefits and outcomes I expect from healthcare?
   - What does "living" mean to me?
   - What does mortality mean?
   - What is quality of life?
   - What do I want for myself in terms of quality and quantity of life?
   - Do I feel entitled to 80-odd years of life? Will I feel cheated if I get less?
   - Do I see death as a failure?

2. To empower past, current, and potential cancer patients to take control of their own health-care by engaging in thought processes that prepare them for the trauma they may experience around a cancer diagnosis.

3. To challenge patients and healthcare providers to think beyond the current model of survivorship care plans after cancer treatment, and to think about the everyday needs of the person, rather than medical convenience.

   This means:

   - seeing the limitations of survivorship care plans (SCPs) as they are currently being used
   - including people with metastatic cancer in our survivorship interventions—those with cancer beyond Stage III are currently not given SCPs, per current mandates
   - acknowledging that patients need help with much more than the current SCP model provides

4. To encourage nurses, physicians, and other professionals to see the importance of interdisciplinary collaboration and reaching out into our communities to complement what we can offer cancer survivors.

References

Kabat-Zinn, J. (2005). *Wherever you go, there you are: Mindfulness meditation in everyday life* (Tenth anniversary edition). New York: Hachette Books.

The details, names, and places in all anecdotes throughout the book have been changed for privacy. I include for legal reasons this disclaimer: This book and its contents, including the Cancer Harbors® and FIERCE: Functional & Fit, Independent, Energized, Restored, Confident, Empowered® programs, are not intended as medical advice or nursing care. For medical advice, consult a licensed physician.

Navigating the C

Contents

Navigating the C

Appendix Contents

Navigating the C

Chapter One: The Survivor Shipwreck

Present-day cancer care

"Compared to what we ought to be, we are only half awake. We are making use of only a small part of our physical and mental resources."
– William James[1]

If you ask me what I do now, I can say several things. I am the cleanup person—I clean up the mess left after cancer treatment. I am also a referee, stepping into a healthcare "game" where all players can benefit from improvement and clarification. Finally, I can also say I'm a closer, a finisher, working to complete the medical system's attempts to restore health.

In these roles, I have the intimate opportunity to witness the suffering, the hope, and the triumphs of the healthcare system. What I see is that both healthcare workers and patients must acknowledge their feelings and humanity. They must stop, reflect inward, and engage in self-care. Those who know what they value, and why, are grounded and resilient in crisis.

Unfortunately, we often do not use our spiritual capabilities to their potential. We are so out of touch with ourselves that we do not think; we just do. Stopping, being, and thinking are not valued as productive uses of time when time is measured in currency.

I came to this perspective as an oncology nurse practicing in traditional healthcare. I now practice in the community. From the outside, my view of cancer care is unobstructed, no longer encased by windowless hospital walls. I see the dysfunction of cancer treatment, from diagnosis to beyond treatment, which leads to waste of time and resources, unnecessary suffering, and poorer outcomes than if we were better connected.

In this chapter, I will lay out three key problems with our current healthcare system's approach to cancer survivorship care. Solving these problems will contribute to better patient outcomes

---

1   McDermott, 1967

and quality of life, as well as decreased healthcare costs. I suggest solving these problems with the qualities of creativity, authenticity, resourcefulness, and empathy, which are so often missing in our current system.

Beginning with a diagnosis of cancer, the healthcare system focuses on *a patient with a disease.* It has little regard for the person and the life he or she had been leading before diagnosis. On our way to curing cancer or putting it in remission, we often do extensive psychological, emotional, social, and functional damage to the patient. We focus on treating a patient with a disease. When the disease is gone, we are left with a patient. Instead, we should be restoring a person.

In cancer care follow-up, there is a push to provide each patient a survivorship care plan (SCP) after treatment (American College of Surgeons Commission on Cancer, 2016). SCPs were developed to address survivors' feelings of being lost after treatment (Institute of Medicine, 2005). But we do not know when is the right time to provide these plans, and we do not offer adequate personal support in conjunction with the plans. We have little data to confirm that SCPs are helping with quality of life, long-term outcomes, costs, or that "lost" feeling (Brennan, Gormally, Butow, Boyle, & Spillane, 2014; Mayer et al., 2014).

The medicalization of cancer survivorship through the use of SCPs can extend the trauma a patient experiences throughout their ordeal with cancer. Even a perfectly-executed SCP does little to restore a patient's sense of self as a separate entity from the medical system. A qualitative definition of *survivorship* should be considered in our medical interventions.

(I use the term survivor to describe a person who has been diagnosed with cancer, from the day of diagnosis, forward, until death. Caregivers and friends may also be included as survivors. Survivorship can be defined as a process that encompasses the health and life of a cancer survivor from diagnosis until death [Wronski, 2015].)[2]

The very term *healthcare* is ill-fitting. It consists of interventions, often physically, psychologically, or emotionally invasive, for the sick. It perpetuates and complicates illness in systems that thrive on that sickness, via medicine and expensive interventions first. Healthcare does not

---

2   A discussion of the history and variation in the terms "cancer survivor" and "cancer survivorship" are contained in Wronski (2015).

focus on self-care to prevent relapse. Healthcare is as sick as the people who come to it.

In healthcare, we have it backward. Treatment consists of medications, invasive procedures, intrusive scans and tests, and needles that draw blood and tissue out of one's body. For too long, services that restore one's function, quality of life, and well-being after disease—such as physical therapy, mental health services, nutrition guidance, and mind-body movement therapies—have been an afterthought or added only if the patient requests them.

In cancer care, the battle mentality dominates. We throw our best chemical and radioactive grenades at the cancer, and the public and media relate to it as an all-out war. These dramatic descriptions contribute to greater public fear of cancer.

Our current treatments—chemotherapy, radiation, surgeries, and others—are the best we have, but they do their own damage. Medicine should complement care, not the other way around.

We in healthcare should provide comfort and restoration during recovery. After cancer treatment is done, patients should be told honestly, "You might be done with treatment, but it's not done with you. There is much more work to do before you are truly finished." *It must be emphasized that this part of care is predominantly under the patient's control.*

We must fix the human elements of the system—the relationships, communication, and respect. When we all are spiritually disconnected, we act as separate beings. We must be accountable to each other, regardless of our place in the system or society. The captain of this ship needs a compass, and the ship must orient itself through meaningful debate, critical thinking, and action by all players in the healthcare system. Everyone who interacts with the healthcare system, from executives to providers, patients, and caregivers, has a role in fixing our broken system.

In present-day healthcare, apathy and risk aversion constrain the executive level and permeate the entire system:

Assumptions are numerous. For example, we assume that people who run businesses are qualified to make decisions about healthcare services. We also assume that the scientific method holds us accountable to better medicine and safety, when the entire process is corruptible with industry conflicts of interest. We assume that new scientific discoveries are being incorporated into current practice. In reality, the entire process—from conducting research studies to reporting results, educating clinicians, and implementing changes in clinical applications to patients—takes decades.

There is little transparency. Most discussions about healthcare policy at the government and organization levels are held behind closed doors. Administrators in healthcare organizations spend too much time in self-congratulatory huddles, celebrating the attainment of "metrics" that don't improve patients' quality of life or relieve their suffering. The mystery around pricing and payment for drugs and services contributes to the precarious financial burden borne by patients, and it threatens our economy.

Talk is insubstantial. The corporate lingo that permeates internal communications and marketing campaigns for healthcare organizations has little substance or inventiveness. Marketing efforts mislead the public, using terms like *precision medicine*, *targeted treatments*, and *personalized care*. The public is encouraged to believe that treatments will be targeted to their individual bodies, when in reality this is not the case.

There is little advancement. Groupthink and risk aversion dominate the healthcare business landscape, new or unconventional ideas are dismissed, and critics are rejected or removed. The production model of healthcare values panacea, process, productivity, and profit over people.

At the provider/patient level of healthcare:

Assumptions are numerous. For example, we assume that death is something to worry about later, cancer is something that happens to someone else, and we are going to live 80 years and then die a painless death in our sleep. People assume the healthcare industry will take care of them when they are sick, without having to direct their own decisions, preparation, and recovery.

In the doctor's office, clinical staff assume their efforts to educate patients are adequate when they have checked the appropriate boxes in the electronic chart, but patients need translations from "medicalese" to practical lay terms. This is work for which nurses are ideally suited. However, nurses must educate patients on the fly because they lack time, staffing, and resources to translate medical jargon effectively.

There is little commitment to changing lifestyle. Despite knowing that exercise, healthy eating, reducing stress, and adopting other positive habits will lower the likelihood of serious or chronic illness, obesity and Type II diabetes are still commonplace. Shiny objects are plentiful. Health fads, products, and services are widely available because their marketing campaigns promise the easy way to health, weight loss, or beauty. In reality, patients need to direct their own healthcare and take responsibility for making decisions, becoming informed, and planning around prevention, self-care, and end-of-life considerations.

There is little awareness. Good health information is drowning in a sea of shoddy information, and many people do not know how to tell the difference. There is a perception that scientific evidence is little more than someone's opinion.

People want hope, but they place hope in the wrong places. They are led astray by marketing campaigns that create feel-good images around cancer care, using tearjerker stories and buzzwords like *patient-centered care* that prey on desperation and lack of understanding.

As we move forward, I see the following three key problems around cancer survivorship. The solutions are inseparable; one cannot be fixed without changing the others.

1. **We must change how we educate healthcare providers and distribute their workloads, allowing them to better serve survivors' needs and concerns.**

   Providing good care takes time, in listening, reflecting, discussing, planning, and evaluating. The distribution of resources to direct patient care and away from administrative work will require a major shift in the healthcare industry as we know it today.

   The high rates of suicide among physicians and burnout among other healthcare providers is evidence of something wrong (Andrew, 2016). They are not machines; they have only so much capacity for volume and pace of work. The unrealistic expectations reduce quality of care and patient outcomes.

   (In this book, the term *healthcare provider* refers to physicians, nurses, and other professionals in healthcare who are credentialed, licensed, and skilled practitioners. There are various schools of thought on the use of the term *provider*, but I am referring to the person inside the white coat or scrubs who provides medical or nursing services and is required to have a license to do so.)

2. **We must improve the public's health literacy, science education, and competence in preventing disease, maintaining health, and managing chronic conditions.**

   Poor health literacy, poor communication, and inadequate time for providers to communicate effectively with patients means that much information shared between provider and patient is not applied to better health outcomes. Instead of placing blind faith in predatory systems that take advantage of short attention spans and easy distractibility, people need to make conscious efforts to focus on, learn about, and practice behavior that is conducive to good health.

3. **Most of all, we must decide if we want to be a health-oriented or a chronic disease-oriented society.**

    This will require introspective thought. We need to ask questions that too few people are asking. We must define health, living, and quality of life for ourselves, *before* we become patients in a healthcare system that is eager to invite us in.

    We must not be afraid to question ourselves and others. When our doctors recommend a treatment, we must ask, "Will this help?" and "What is the likelihood that this will cause unintended effects or interfere with my quality of life?" We should make time for self-reflection, contemplation, and critical thinking. When we clarify our values *before* we get sick, we are less likely to be led down a path we did not intend to choose. When we lack information about what lies along that path, we are more likely to be traumatized.

    Apathy and the lack of civic engagement on matters pertaining to healthcare must be upended. Patients and healthcare professionals alike must insist on representation in policy and legislative matters, must speak out against policies that contribute to greater inequality and reduced access to medical care, and must vote accordingly and with diligence.

    We need a mature, rational approach to matters of health, disease, and mortality. When we wait until we are hit by a shocking diagnosis to think about health, panic and anxiety cloud our minds. Efforts of healthcare providers, attempting to educate us during a crisis, go to waste.

    Death happens to all of us, and accepting that improves the way we live. Health and cancer, and quality of life and cancer, need not be mutually exclusive. Many people can and do have years of quality living with Stage IV (incurable) cancer. They should be seen, heard, and not forgotten in our efforts to improve healthcare for all.

When people are informed, prepared, and have resources to make choices, most choose health and good quality of life. Let's begin by acknowledging and honoring our values, educating ourselves, and initiating conversations with those who help us practice our values.

In this chapter, I have presented what I believe are the primary problems in cancer care today. Before I launch into solutions, however, I will explain how my own path through healthcare led me to this understanding. What I learned along the way steered me to my current work and the reason for this book.

References

American College of Surgeons Commission on Cancer. (2014). Accreditation committee clarifi-cations for standard 3.3 survivorship care plan. Retrieved June 26, 2017, from https://www.facs.org/publications/newsletters/coc-source/special-source/standard33

American College of Surgeons Commission on Cancer. (2016). *Cancer program standards: Ensuring patient-centered care* (2016 Edition). Chicago: Author. Retrieved November 22, 2017, from https://www.facs.org/~/media/files/quality%20programs/cancer/coc/2016%20coc%20stan-dards%20manual_interactive%20pdf.ashx

Andrew, L. B. (2016). Physician suicide. Retrieved March 20, 2017, from http://emedicine.medscape.com/article/806779-overview

Brennan, M. E., Gormally, J. F., Butow, P., Boyle, F. M., & Spillane, A. J. (2014). Survivorship care plans in cancer: A systematic review of care plan outcomes. *British Journal of Cancer, 111*(10), 1899-1908. doi:10.1038/bjc.2014.505

Institute of Medicine and National Research Council. (2005). From cancer patient to cancer sur-vivor: Lost in transition. Washington, D.C.: The National Academies Press. doi:10.17226/11468

Mayer, D. K., Nekhlyudov, L., Snyder, C. F., Merrill, J. K., Wollins, D. S., & Shulman, L. N. (2014). American Society of Clinical Oncology clinical expert statement on cancer survivorship care planning. *Journal of Oncology Practice, 10*(6), 345-351. doi:10.1200/JOP.2014.001321

McDermott, J. J. (Ed.). (1967). *The writings of William James: A comprehensive edition*. New York: Random House.

Wronski, S. L. (2015). Defining cancer survivor and cancer survivorship: The who, what, and when. *Psicooncologia, 12*(1), 7-18. doi:10.5209/rev_PSIC.2015.v12.n1.48900

Chapter Two: Between Drift and Full Sail

The author's experience with healthcare

"The important thing is not to stop questioning."

– Albert Einstein[1]

My first run-in with cancer was in 1966, when I was two years old, but I was unaware of it. My paternal grandfather died of acute myeloid leukemia that year, at 48 years old. I remember him lying on the couch at their row house in northeast Philadelphia, his face very pale. I wanted to approach him but my grandmother told me not to.

My grandmother wouldn't tell anyone, not even her kids, about his cancer until he was on his deathbed, hemorrhaging from the leukemia. My dad still recounts this with visible frustration at the secrecy my grandmother kept.

In those days, cancer was kept quiet, talked about in whispers, as if it were something shameful. Several years later, one of my maternal great-aunts was diagnosed with breast cancer at age 40, and I remember my grandmother and her sisters whispering about her at a family gathering.

As a child, I attended both public elementary school and Quaker school, but my early values and beliefs were established in Quaker school. It exposed me to critical thought and ideas I would not have encountered in public school, such as the history of conscientious objection. The Quaker values of social and economic justice, equal human rights, and responsible stewardship of resources stayed with me despite my non-religious personal leaning.

In junior high, my parents divorced. I moved from Philadelphia to Scottsdale, Arizona, with my dad and new stepmom before I began public high school in 1978. To my 14-year-old eyes, I

---

1   Old Man's Advice to Youth: "Never Lose a Holy Curiosity," 1955, p. 64

might as well have moved to another planet. I could see the sky, and the air was so clear it was possible to see fifty or more miles away. I was fascinated by the desert and joined the backpacking club right away.

The western cliffs of the Superstition Mountains were visible from the cotton fields east of our house near the Salt River Pima-Maricopa Indian Community. I spent many weekends and long school vacations hiking far into the Superstition Wilderness.

During my senior year in college at Northern Arizona University, where I majored in forestry, I started running for fitness. I enjoyed it and was good at it so after graduation, I became a competitive runner in road races. Eventually I started running ultramarathons (distances of 100 miles or more). Five years after college graduation, I found myself in graduate school at Colorado State University. I started a master's in exercise physiology program but soon realized it didn't resonate with my true interests. Thinking of my background in natural resources, on a whim I approached the department chair in recreation resources. From that day forward, I pursued a doctorate in the benefits of leisure, combining my interests in the physiology of exercise with the psychophysiological health benefits of outdoor leisure experiences.

In 1994, I graduated with a Doctor of Philosophy in recreation resources. I took a temporary faculty position at a small college, teaching exercise science and health promotion classes. I loved teaching, but I was not suited to the academic world. For a few years, I struggled to find a new direction. My husband and I moved back to Arizona in 1998 to pursue opportunities closer to my family. I started a personal training business working with women over age 40 who experienced chronic health conditions, such as autoimmune diseases with symptoms of fatigue and chronic joint pain. These women were unable to participate in regular exercise programs or work with trainers who did not understand their physical limitations.

My clients wanted to exercise, but they had no idea how to create a safe and effective training program. They needed someone to guide them while taking into consideration their individual needs. I researched their conditions and their medications to determine what precautions they needed to take, and I developed light exercise training programs to prevent debilitating soreness or injuries.

During this experience, I learned what my clients were missing in their medical care—that exercise and healthy behaviors could fill a gaping hole to improve their quality of life. Unfortunately, many of their doctors did not suggest exercise and often had nothing more to offer than additional medications.

I enjoyed the creative process of educating my clients on taking care of themselves, but I realized I could be even more effective if I had a medical background. I would understand the rationale behind their doctors' recommendations, and I could help them get the most out of their self-care efforts.

There was talk of a nursing shortage, and hospitals would pay for nursing school, requiring little commitment after graduation. Once the furthest thing from my mind, nursing seemed like a good idea.

Headwind

Some years before this, starting in my early 30s, I became aware of an odd pattern in my health. I would feel exceptionally good for several months, having a lot of energy and feeling superb. Then, over a few more months, I would slow down, feel sluggish, gain weight, and want to sleep all the time. I felt depressed and couldn't focus on mental tasks. Over a few years, I cycled back and forth. It seemed to get worse and more extreme with each swing. I started having heart palpitations, hot flashes, and mood swings, and then I would cycle back to wanting to sleep most of the day. I lacked enough concentration to even read the newspaper. I wanted to apply to nursing school, but I couldn't study in my condition.

My running also suffered. I had always been one of the faster runners, and it wasn't unusual for me to win races. Now, people twenty and thirty years older were beating me. When I tried to run, I felt like I had elephant legs. I wanted to lie down and sleep at the side of the road.

All I wanted was to feel normal, have a working brain, and enjoy running again.

While describing my condition to a friend, she suggested I have my thyroid checked. My TSH (thyroid stimulating hormone, an indicator of thyroid function) levels were found to be elevated. My doctor felt a possible goiter in my neck and referred me to an endocrinologist. It took three months to get an appointment.

The first endocrinologist was abrasive, and I got the feeling she thought I was wasting her time. She literally tossed a package of medication samples across the examining table at me, told me to get rechecked in six to eight weeks, and left the room.

I took the medication but immediately started looking for another endocrinologist. Over many months, I saw several endocrinologists, who each made minor changes to my medication. One doctor discovered I had Hashimoto's thyroiditis, a common autoimmune disease of the thyroid. My TSH lab values came down into the normal range, but I didn't feel much better. I was sleeping less, but I continued to have problems focusing and thinking clearly.

Nearly two years after my family doctor first checked my thyroid, I wondered if I was stuck with this nonfunctional brain as a permanent condition. Nursing school was still out of the question. I wondered if I would ever run again without feeling like my legs were stuck in concrete. Running competitively, which I loved, was not possible, as I needed mental sharpness to maintain the intensity of training and racing.

The Healthcare Heretic

I began searching the Internet for answers to my health conditions, finding chat groups and information websites. I also searched for another doctor who might take a different approach to my thyroid problems. Finally I found one in Phoenix. It took another three months to get an appointment, but she was well-recommended by the strangers I chatted with online.

She was my fifth doctor, and she was focused and thorough. She asked questions none of the other doctors had. She asked how I felt when I was running and when I was trying to read. She wanted to know how my health was affecting my life. She asked what I wanted out of this visit.

I told her I wanted to be able to use my brain, and I wanted to run ultramarathons again. I could not remember any other time a doctor had asked me questions like these. She spent a full hour with me, studied my labs, and discussed the Hashimoto's disease process. She also told me she was a thyroid cancer survivor.

She learned that everyone feels best at different levels of thyroid hormone replacement. The TSH lab values that were considered the normal range were under debate by endocrinologists, and she preferred to focus on how the patient was feeling instead of the lab values.

The key was not expecting what works for one person to work for another person. She understood that I was in tune with my body as an athlete and a person educated in the health sciences, as well as a person who valued my physical and mental well-being.

At the end she made only a minor change to my treatment, adding a second medication. Within a week I noticed I was thinking clearly again. I began to feel better on my runs.

Not long after, I decided to enter a local trail marathon, my first race in two years. I felt great; I felt like a runner again. With my health returning to normal, I applied to nursing school.

Adrift

I do not know why the other endocrinologists and doctors were unable to recommend this new medication sooner. I do know, however, that the doctors had not asked how my thyroid imbalance was affecting my life. They did not listen to me; they treated me off the lab numbers and nothing else. When my descriptions of my symptoms did not agree with the labs, they classified me as a perimenopausal woman and tried to treat me for anxiety and depression instead of looking further.

In this moment, I realized how healthcare could be improved. I understood firsthand what my personal training clients had been telling me. They were not being heard. Their health conditions or diseases were being treated, but they weren't being restored to good health. There was more to treating a disease than eradicating the pathophysiological process. Treatment needed to start with questions leading to an individualized approach.

I wasn't sure how this understanding would manifest in my work, but I moved forward with nursing school. Somehow, I knew that on the other side of nursing there was a path to doing something with these valuable insights.

Before I began school, I worked as a certified nursing assistant (CNA) in a hospital medical and oncology unit. I didn't choose oncology; it was what was available. I wanted to know what I was getting into, and the hospital would pay my tuition when I started school.

As I worked, I observed all aspects of oncology: breaking the news of cancer, the psychological impacts on patients from diagnosis through treatment or end-of-life, various medical procedures, and the tragic deaths of young patients. My interest was piqued, and my eyes were opened with every shift.

Low Tide

Entering nursing school at age 41 was a bit of a shock. I wasn't the only middle-aged person in class; it seemed that more than half of us were starting a new career. Academically, nursing school was easy. It felt like a lot of busywork after a Ph.D. program heavy in physiology and statistics. I learned the most by observing during my clinical assignments.

No matter what facility I was in, I noticed that the nurses ran from room to room, giving medications, printing off forms, and trying to offload work to the CNAs. They rarely took lunch or bathroom breaks. I learned right away that I needed to keep a snack in my side pocket if I was to make it through a shift standing up. I would stuff a bite in my mouth whenever I had clean hands and thirty seconds to chew without having to talk to someone. Finding those 30 seconds was a challenge.

Waitresses on Roller Skates

For patients, I imagined that a stay in the hospital was like being kept in a zoo. As they would wait for the physician to issue orders for further evaluation or discharge, nurses, nursing assistants, physical therapists, and countless others would cycle through their rooms around the clock.

Ideally, care would have been coordinated among the numerous staff involved in treating a patient. The nursing assistant would have changed the bedsheets while the patient was in physical therapy, or the nurse would have given the patient pain medication before the therapist arrived, but it never went that smoothly. No one knew what the other department's schedule was; no planning or communication occurred among any of the staff.

There was noise, artificial light, hard linoleum floors, cold rooms, and little comfort except when visited by family.

When a patient was declared ready to go home, a nurse began the lengthy discharge paperwork process, knowing that the moment the patient was gone, another patient would be admitted and the labor-intensive process would start all over again.

It seemed like a factory production line, yet there was little healing involved. Patients' symptoms were abated, but they left the hospital without the skills to avoid readmission for recurrence of the same illness.

Observing this as a student, I occasionally wondered why we were trained to understand pathophysiology and pharmacology when it appeared that nurses were little more than overworked waitstaff. It seemed nurses were not used in accordance with their knowledge and skill and that their training was underutilized in the constant rush of menial tasks. Another nurse described it as being a "waitress on roller skates."

Of course, nurses have great responsibility for patients' safety throughout their entire stay. Nurses must understand disease processes, diagnoses, symptoms, treatments, medications, side effects, and so much more. And they do it—twelve hours or more each day, on their feet, often with no breaks even to use the bathroom.

After my final extended clinical experience in the cardiovascular ICU on the night shift, I graduated nursing school. Bracing myself, I sought my first job. I knew it wouldn't be easy, but I told myself, *This is a skill I will always have, as well as a potential source of income to support myself.*

I could hear my instructors saying, "Nursing has so many opportunities. You can do almost anything with nursing. If you don't like one type of nursing, you can move into something else."

Parking Garage Prayers

I took my first nursing job in a medical-neurosurgical intensive care unit. I had heard mixed opinions from other nurses about entering the ICU as a new graduate. Some said it was too hard and that I should gain experience first in a medical-surgical unit. Others acknowledged the difficulties but said it could be done, stressing it would require multiple years to feel comfortable.

In most hospital settings, there are neither training resources nor enough patient, empathetic, and willing people to guide a new graduate to comfort as an ICU nurse. Instead, new nurses typically incur significant emotional trauma during their early career years.

A few weeks before I started my new job, my younger sister was diagnosed with breast cancer. She was 35 and had a 2-year-old son. At the time we were unaware of a family history of breast cancer, but our mother finally told us then about our great aunt's experience with breast cancer.

My sister opted for bilateral mastectomy with reconstruction for her Stage I, estrogen-receptor positive cancer. Despite my status as a new employee, I was allowed to take time off and spend a few days with her after her surgery.

Starting work in the ICU was a whirlwind of learning and feeling overwhelmed. I could get through a shift, but I was physically and mentally drained at the end.

I worked weekends as much as possible because the more experienced nurses worked then. They were highly skilled, secure in their knowledge, and unlikely to lash out at a new nurse for asking a question or feeling uncertain. Their confidence and efficiency allowed them more energy to mentor a new nurse.

Two years into it, however, I still did not feel comfortable. I learned to watch my back with several coworkers because it was common to find a knife in it. Depending on who was working on a given day, a crisis situation could go very well, or very poorly and stressfully.

One day I put a blood pressure cuff on my arm in an empty room. It read 160/101. Me, a 120-pound endurance athlete. Over time, though, I figured out which nurses I could rely on in a bad situation, and we helped each other out.

I realized it was not the patient care stressing me out, but rather the demeanor of a few of my fellow nurses—and occasionally the doctors, who had the authority to make my life miserable. I was depressed, and at times I felt barely functional enough to untangle IV tubing around a patient.

I am not a religious person, but each morning when I pulled into the parking garage, I would recite the Peace Prayer of St. Francis. I prayed to myself, the universe, or whatever was out there to help me not hurt anyone.

"Lord, make me an instrument of your peace:
Where there is hatred, let me sow love;
Where there is injury, pardon;
Where there is doubt, faith;
Where there is despair, hope;
Where there is darkness, light;
Where there is sadness, joy.
Grant that I may not so much seek
To be consoled as to console, to be understood as to understand, to be loved as to love..."
– from the Peace Prayer of St. Francis

Help me be peaceful, help me not lose my mind, help me not throttle the charge nurse, I recited day after day.

Nearly all of the pulmonologists, who were the ICU doctors, were nice to work with and helpfully explained the rationale behind their decisions. Most of the hospitalists and other specialty physicians who came to the ICU were helpful, too. But the worst doctor I worked with was a former nurse who became a physician. She clicked her heels as she walked around the ICU with a look of disgust on her face.

Once I approached her about something my patient needed urgently. I broke into her conversation with another physician, asserting myself as delicately as I could. She turned to me and yelled in my face, "I'll get to it when I have time!"

The physician next to her kept a blank look on her face. I felt my face turning red. It was the last straw for me. At that moment, I was done. I knew I needed to leave the ICU. I had been withstanding abuse for too long, and I wasn't getting anywhere professionally. I wasn't learning skills other than assisting with invasive procedures, giving cardiac medications, and running codes, mostly on patients who were not fully conscious.

I needed two-way human interaction and to escape an environment so punishing, demanding, and unsupportive for me. It was completely at odds with healing and quality of life for patients.

Rain

In late 2009, I road-tripped with my friend Katy to run a race on the Hopi reservation in northern Arizona. The wide-open skies and vistas of the high desert were a relief from the chaotic environment at work.

After the race and a great weekend, we started back home. We were stopped at a gas station when my phone rang.

It was my dad. He asked if I could talk and if I was sitting down. He then told me he'd been diagnosed with a rare type of chronic leukemia. I knew chronic leukemia was not as immediately life-threatening as acute leukemia, but that was all I knew. I could hear the worry in my dad's voice. I imagined he was thinking of his own father's death nearly 50 years earlier.

I hid the tears in my voice until I got off the phone with him. I wanted to turn the car around and drive directly to my dad in Phoenix instead of home to Colorado, but I couldn't wrap my head around it. Katy drove us back to Colorado, while I researched what I could on my phone when we had a connection.

At that point, his doctors were not recommending treatment. It would be a watching and waiting process. As I found out more, I discovered that my dad had been feeling poorly for some time. He had been anemic, had swollen lymph nodes, and was prone to upper respiratory infections. I could remember thinking that he had been getting a lot of colds. The last time I had seen him I thought he looked different, but I couldn't put my finger on it then. After his diagnosis I realized his pallor and swollen lymph nodes were symptoms I knew well from my time in the oncology unit. It hadn't occurred to me when I was looking at my own father.

As it turned out, my dad's labs had shown a gradual worsening of anemia and neutropenia over several years, but his primary care doctor had not noticed. Shortly thereafter, his doctor revealed he had dementia, gave up his license, and closed his practice.

The outcome of my dad's treatment might not have changed had the anemia and neutropenia been noted earlier, but it certainly would have helped my dad understand why he was so tired. He may have avoided infections and overworking himself during that time.

Moving the Compass

After learning of my dad's leukemia, I started looking for a new job, this time in oncology. I also began attending cancer support meetings to learn how to support my dad. It took nine more months, but I eventually landed a job in outpatient oncology.

I adjusted easily to my new job. The patients were not sedated, as they often were in the ICU, so they could communicate what they wanted. They went home after their appointments. My tasks were specialized but basic, with little urgency: check orders for chemotherapy, rule out contraindications to treatment, assess the patient for adverse effects, contact the oncologist with any concerns, and communicate with the lab and pharmacy.

The Missing Pieces

While making my patients comfortable, doing the physical assessment, and giving medications, there was time to talk. Mostly I left the talking to the patient and just listened. Over and over I heard concerns and questions that had been unaddressed: information that would have im-proved the patient's comfort, safety, or tolerance of their treatment regimen.

I wondered, *How could no one have discussed this with the patient?* It was apparent to me that treatment was interfering with their lifestyles. What would happen after they completed treatment? What would their lives would be like when we no longer saw them regularly, after their hair grew back, and when they were expected to return to their lives as they were before the shock of a cancer diagnosis?

During this time, I continued attending the cancer support meetings, wanting to learn whether there was a better way to help cancer survivors with their unmet needs. What I witnessed opened my eyes. Survivors were happy with their doctors' care, but the lasting effects of treatment were interfering with their return to normal activities. In many cases, their entire lives had been upended. They were unsure when they would feel better, or *if* they would ever feel better.

Once again I saw the focus on medical interventions over lifestyle, just as I had a dozen or so years earlier with my personal training clients. I also remembered my experience as a thyroid patient: how my treatment as a number interfered with my ideal level of functioning. I might always have thyroid problems, but at least I could feel good enough to forget about it most of the time. For patients with cancer, this seemed less likely.

It wasn't that doctors did not care, but they had been trained to think one way, and their time constraints limited what they were able to provide. For me, it took a doctor who made time to help *after* treatment as much as she did during treatment. The system is not set up to accommodate that time, however.

Patients are under-informed and unprepared for what life will be like after treatment. They are so grateful to their doctors for saving their lives that they often avoid asserting their own needs in follow-up appointments. Older patients, who are the majority of cancer patients, especially want to please their doctor and do not readily open up about everyday fatigue or functional difficulties. They get swept into the doctor's agenda of quick, efficient follow-up appointments unless the doctor is attuned to the patient's needs.

Facing Mortality

The most troubling gap in communication was when the patient had a poor prognosis and had little time left, especially when recently diagnosed with advanced cancer. Few doctors seemed comfortable talking to patients and their family members about death and its imminence. Further, few patients seemed prepared for death even when palliative treatment was being used only to relieve symptoms and there was no chance of achieving a cure or remission.

As a nurse, among the most frustrating experiences is giving a patient chemotherapy when it will not result in better quality of life. Instead, it often extends the patient's sick time, and he or she is less able to enjoy their remaining time on earth with their loved ones.

Too many times, I witnessed a patient with very advanced cancer receive a chemotherapy infusion, get markedly worse, be admitted to the hospital, and die shortly thereafter. This usually happened when patients and their families refused to give up hope, were misinformed, or were in denial, despite overwhelming and imminent signs of death. It also happened occasionally when doctors and nurses, uncomfortable with discussing death with a patient, gave false hope or withheld information the patient needed to make decisions about end-of-life plans. The patients, or their families, could not recognize the futility of further treatment, denying them the comfort-focused care of hospice.

The Importance of CARE

Nurses see patients more frequently and for longer periods of time than physicians. They see them when they enter the hospital or the infusion center. They know when patients are not feeling well, and they watch their conditions progress. Nurses are trusted, deservedly so, because they have the skills, knowledge, and understanding that are critical to communication during the rush of a medical appointment.

The acronym CARE—creativity, authenticity, resourcefulness, and empathy—emphasizes qualities that nurses bring to the patient experience. Nurses understand the disease process, medications, and their benefits and risks. They are experts on the effects of disease on a person's well-being.

Helping cancer survivors restore quality of life after treatment requires skill and a focus on empathy. It is holistic in its approach. Nurses are the ideal professionals to lead this change.

As I sat in on support group meetings and patient conversations, I realized that with my background in health, recreation, and wellness, along with my clinical nursing experience, I was in an ideal position to address these issues.

Pulling Up Anchors

The culture of healthcare in the U.S. in 2013 reflected the major changes taking place at the time: megamergers, executive musical chairs, and turbulence throughout the entire system.

Among healthcare executives there was an aversion to creativity, innovation, and risk. Staff and management were rewarded for maintaining the status quo. The qualities of creativity, authenticity, resourcefulness, and empathy were often forced out of nurses through rigorous, mind-numbing overwork. Nurses are expected to keep the machine running smoothly; they're expected not to make waves.

Unable to contain my frustration at the system that was so unwilling to risk innovation, I was determined to come up with a better way to help people restore their quality of life after cancer.

I left the hospital and began to write educational materials to answer to patients' most common questions. I took on the role of a health coach and started a combined movement class and support group for cancer survivors.

I named the class FIERCE, for Functional & Fit, Independent, Energized, Restored, Confident, Empowered. The class encompassed all those concepts—not just the physical aspect of recovery, but also enjoyment of movement, variety, learning, socializing, and the health benefits derived from those activities.

FIERCE began in October 2014 with three participants. It has been growing ever since.

Next, I developed a program named Cancer Harbors. The phrase, "Because living is so much more than surviving," became its *raison d'être*—its reason for being. The content addresses the specific issues that kept arising among my patients with various cancers. It helps survivors manage the lasting physical, emotional, and functional effects of treatment that continue to impact their quality of life.

The program attempts to solve several problems. First, patients need help with self-care skills after treatment. Survivorship care plans were not addressing their quality of life needs, instead serving as follow-up medical screening. Fear and anxiety about recurrence plagued survivors constantly, along with ongoing and unrelieved fatigue. There was no one to address their everyday coping skills, physically or psychologically. Only those with excellent health literacy and self-advocacy skills persisted when their needs were not met.

Second, survivors need help getting referrals to a multitude of additional services, such as physical and occupational therapy, relaxation and mind-body/movement therapies, exercise coaching and guidance, nutrition counseling, massage therapy, peer support, mental health, relationship counseling, sex therapy, and many more. These services that survivors needed were unaffordable, unavailable locally, or unknown to them. Most doctors and nurses were equally unaware of the community providers who could help. There was no collaboration, referral system, or cost coverage to ensure continuity of recovery after medical intervention.

Third, the program helps survivors clarify their values around the quality of their lives—that is, how do they achieve the quality of life they want? They need guidance in defining those values and encouragement to allow their values to lead them down their path to recovery. They need help finding the trailhead for their personal path to recovery, and they need help staying on their path.

Everyone I had known and listened to over the years about cancer treatment—the people in the cancer support groups I attended for years, people in the community, my old personal training clients, my family members—all said surviving was not enough.

Despite having highly trained and skilled experts in patient care, the healthcare system was failing patients. Doctors and nurses were putting cancer into remission, but they didn't know what would happen later.

Patients were done with treatment, for now. The problem was, treatment wasn't done with them.

References

Old Man's Advice to Youth: "Never Lose a Holy Curiosity." (May 2, 1955). *Life, 38*(18). Retrieved November 17, 2017, from https://books.google.com/books?id=dlYEAAAAMBAJ&lpg=PP1&dq=Life%2C%202%20May%201955&pg=PA61#v=snippet&q=questioning&f=false

Chapter Three: Atlas Drowned

Improving physician culture and cancer care

"Stress is an epidemic in our country..."

– Vivek Murthy, 19th Surgeon General of the United States[1]

We all experience illness and see a physician at some point in our lives. Physicians are the main orchestrators of a return to health, and rightly so. They apply the science of medicine to diagnose, treat, and cure disease. For this reason, they have long enjoyed a high regard in the United States. In past generations, physicians were almost deified, a combination of paternalism and omniscience that were accepted and even taken for granted. Patients expected the doctor to tell them what to do and were unlikely to question a doctor's recommendations.

In the case of a cancer diagnosis, patients' fear of cancer makes them vulnerable in the care of the oncologists whose advice they seek. This vulnerability endures beyond cancer treatment and can affect patients for the rest of their lives. Because of this great responsibility, oncologists' and other physicians' care is critical to a patient's quality of life outcome after cancer.

In this chapter I discuss how physician culture impacts their care of cancer patients. Then I discuss qualities of good cancer care and how to overcome some of the shortcomings in physician culture and cancer care.

This chapter is written from my point of view as a nurse, based on what I have observed in hospital, outpatient, and community settings. My intent here is not to blame physicians for shortcomings in cancer care; I am simply pointing out what I see and suggesting solutions for improvement. When I refer to "physicians" I am talking not only about oncologists, but all doctors who work with cancer patients.

---

1   Cox, 2016

Physician Preparation, Stresses, and Work Culture

Preparation for a career in medicine requires and reinforces certain characteristics. The training is mentally and physically rigorous, and the demand for high academic performance favors those who are perfectionists, compulsive, competitive, and objective (Lipsenthal, 2009).

Medical school indoctrinates students into the medical culture, honing these characteristics even further. Long hours of studying, clinical experiences, and residencies demand that students sacrifice social interactions. They may become disconnected and isolated from their peers. The teaching and learning styles favor memorization, facts, multiple choice testing, objective evaluation, and hands-on learning experience.

Medical school, internships, and residencies can be almost military-like in their demands and have been described as abusive (TEDMED, 2016) and paternalistic, especially in settings where older physicians with traditional attitudes are in command. The American Medical Association (AMA) has been described even by themselves as having characteristics of conservatism (Pho, 2011) and paternalism (American Medical Association, 2004). Lisa S. Bliss, MD, a solo practicing physiatrist (physical medicine and rehabilitation) in Spokane, Washington, said that residents have been required to work while ill, even expected to complete their rounds while receiving IV fluids, because it was done that way in the past. Doctors would say, "That's the way I did it" (personal communication, March 31, 2017).

Many physicians suffer from a great deal of stress. They work long hours, sacrificing family, social, and community connections. They often do not get enough regular physical activity, leisure time, or sleep, especially when they are on call or work many days in a row. Adequate nutrition is a challenge, as spacing, timing, and content of meals may be determined by each day's events. Additionally, they may have financial stress from medical school debt and other necessary expenses such as malpractice insurance, maintenance of certifications, and continuing education.

Physicians also face continual pressure to make the right decisions in life-or-death situations, they witness raw emotions of patients and family members when they give bad news, and they are present for the deaths of patients.

These stressors and traumas take their toll, but physicians have no established standards of self-care or restorative activities built into their work culture. They simply move from one difficult case to another and are expected to bury their feelings to remain focused and objective. Debriefing or counseling after a grueling experience is not part of their work plan.

Physicians may feel pressure to not be seen taking breaks or engaging in self-care on work-days. Dr. Bliss felt for a long time that she could not leave the office dressed in her cycling gear, as she did not want anyone to question why she was not working. Over time she has become more comfortable with her peers, but she still does not allow patients to see her in bike gear (personal communication, March 31, 2017).

Diagnoses of major depression, anxiety, bipolar disorder, or other mental illness—even antide-pressant use—is subject to scrutiny and penalty by the licensing boards. Even if a physician is functioning well, the licensing boards may take a punitive approach. The burden of proof is on the physician to demonstrate he or she is competent to serve. This discourages many doctors from seeking treatment for stress or mental illness.

Medical culture simply does not allow doctors to be human and acknowledge emotions or their need for help. The inability to resolve emotional stress around work has led to high rates of suicide among physicians (Andrew, 2016).

Over the past decade, the adoption of the electronic health record, along with changes in regulations and the way physicians are reimbursed under healthcare reform, have led to the closing of numerous private practices. Many physicians are now employed by large healthcare corporations.

These physicians are subject to the demands of healthcare administrators who prioritize cost savings, maximizing profits, and growing the organization. Healthcare administrators may have little understanding of the impact of short appointments, patient satisfaction scores, and restric-tions on physicians' autonomy and function in the patient-physician relationship.

The demands of working for large organizations can pressure doctors into satisfying patients even when they demand treatment that is inappropriate for their condition. Many physicians feel pressure to keep patient satisfaction scores high to keep their jobs.

In addition to the pressures of working for large corporations, physicians must also fight faceless insurance companies to cover care they recommend for their patients. For many physicians, the worst part of the job is fighting insurance company denials for care. Dr. Bliss said insurance companies are an "invisible god of healthcare who says you can't do this for your patient." She never takes the denials personally because she knows what she's doing. "You can't see who you're fighting, and when they deny it, they don't tell you why or what you need to do differently to get it accepted, how to fix it" (personal communication, March 31, 2017).

Disincentives to becoming a doctor (Kavilanz, 2009), including lower pay and reimbursements, less autonomy in practice as an employee of a healthcare corporation, and the ability to earn more as an administrator or executive have led to physician shortages in some specialties, including oncology (National Academy of Sciences, 2009). Further, the debt and pressures of medical school, combined with paternalism, drill sergeant-like tactics, and the self-sacrificial work culture of physicians, has led to an epidemic of suicide and burnout among physicians (TEDMED, 2016).

A more collaborative, supportive, and realistic approach is needed. A high quality of life for doctors and their patients, placing self-care as a priority, should be valued. Doctors should not be expected to transcend their own humanity. They are human and need compassion—not just for their patients, but for themselves.

How the Medical Approach Impacts Cancer Care and Outcomes

Wherever medical treatment is applied, there is always the potential for unintended harm. Iatrogenesis is the "inadvertent and preventable induction of disease or complications by the medical treatment or procedures of a physician or surgeon" (Merriam-Webster, n.d.).

In cancer treatment, the entire process of care from diagnosis onward offers a host of treatments that are hard on the body, creating iatrogenic trauma that impacts mental and emotional health. Informed consent is designed to educate patients about the risks and benefits of any procedure, which is the medical professional's duty and is required by law. Many physicians readily admit that their treatments can cause harm (Brawley, 2011) and that there is a tradeoff for medical interventions. The more invasive and complicated an intervention, generally, the greater the risk—for example, a double mastectomy for breast cancer and the effect it has on a woman's sexuality. The damage done ranges from minimal to severe impact on the patient's quality of life or survival, and can be physical, functional, or psychosocial in nature.

* * *

The following are examples of typical harm in cancer care that I have observed.

1) Prostate cancer treatment has long done more harm than good when men are over-treated. Radiation, hormone treatments, and radical prostatectomy all create serious quality of life issues for men who undergo them. Consequences may include erectile dysfunction, incontinence, damage to the colon and rectum, and depletion of testosterone. There are grave emotional and psychological consequences for the patient, as well as significant impact on their relationships.

Men are often not informed that radiation damage progresses even after treatment is complete, and they may experience harm that is only evident months to years later. Men (and women as well) are not often referred to physical therapists for education on pelvic floor strengthening, or to sex therapists to improve sexual and intimacy concerns. Both patients and doctors are uncomfortable discussing these topics, but doctors must do so to support the patient's quality of life.

2) A patient with end-stage lung cancer was referred to a large academic center for a clinical trial about an hour's drive from her home. She arrived at the center to receive a lung biopsy. Thinking she would go home the next day, she arrived with a friend who could help her for the day. During the biopsy, she experienced a collapsed lung and was stuck in the hospital for days with a painful chest tube to re-inflate her lung. She had to make new arrangements for someone to pick her up. She had been unaware something like this could happen. It was described in the informed consent, but she did not understand what it meant.

3) The oncologist treating a patient with Stage IV cancer did not recommend further treatment, except palliative measures. The last PET scan revealed scattered small lesions in the brain, but the patient and accompanying family member were not informed. Shortly after, the patient began to experience loss of balance, but thought it was unrelated to the cancer since she was not receiving treatment. When she suddenly began vomiting a week later, she saw her oncologist's partner, who sent her immediately for brain irradiation. The patient was shocked and upset to learn the cancer had spread to her brain. She wished she had been told about the brain metastases so she could have been alert for the symptoms and sought relief sooner.

4) A woman with Stage III ovarian cancer underwent primary treatment of surgery and chemotherapy. The oncologist did not discuss with her and her husband the likelihood of recurrence. After a clear PET scan, the couple thought the cancer was behind them. Eight months later, however, she experienced a bowel obstruction and ureteral blockage, and it was found the

cancer had returned. The news left them feeling angry, distraught, and betrayed by the treatment team. They suspected the doctors lied to them. They delayed further treatment seeking a different opinion, only to be told the same thing by each doctor: that it is not unusual for ovarian cancer to recur.

One could argue the patients suffered no true harm in these experiences, but harm is not only determined by life or death. Quality of life and trust in their medical team was negatively affected for these patients, and these consequences were of great importance.

Slipping Through the Cracks in Cancer Patient Care

Inconsistency in communication and supportive follow-up care is common. There is often a disconnect between the information doctors intend to convey to their patients and what the patient hears (Barnlund, 1970). This is caused by patient anxiety, low health literacy, feeling overwhelmed, feeling unwell, and numerous other factors.

Communication

Several critical events in patient care provide openings for miscommunication, with some of the most common described below.

> *Cancer diagnosis* – Cancer diagnosis causes emotional trauma, and patients live with anxiety for the rest of their lives. Because they are so fearful of cancer, they respond with anxiety and paralysis and are unable to process information they receive from their doctors. Patients should always have an advocate with them to help record information.
> In these situations, patients often want their doctor to tell them what to do. They do not always seek a second opinion, even when it would be wise to do so. Patients should understand that there is not always a single correct answer, but that treatment decisions could affect their quality of life later.
>
> Doctors should ensure that the uninformed, anxious, newly-diagnosed patient receives counseling and education from nurses, social workers, and mental health providers. Patients should understand they have time to make decisions and should learn about the benefits, risks, and long-term consequences of all options, including not treating. Patients should not make sudden decisions, as a cancer diagnosis rarely requires emergency action.

Discussing outcomes of treatment – The patient and family should understand what outcome is likely after treatment. Physicians must ensure their treatment goals are aligned with the patient's, and that the goals are mutually understood before proceeding.

Doctors should convey clearly when they administer treatment palliatively—to manage symptoms without expectation of remission, recovery, or cure. When not fully explained, palliative treatment[2] can provide false hope to a family and patient who expect to achieve a cure or prolong life.

Discussing remission, recurrence, and risk – Doctors must explain the differences between absolute risk, relative risk, overall survival, progression-free survival, and other metrics from research on the recommended treatment. (These terms are discussed in the Cancer Harbors module titled "Prevention, Risk & Cause" available at https://cancerharbors.com/table-of-contents-cancer-harbors/.)

Doctors frequently overestimate the benefits of treatment and underestimate the risks (Hoffmann & Del Mar, 2017). Therefore, doctors should make great effort to objectively convey to their patients survival rates and times for treatment versus non-treatment; for example, patients should be informed if a certain treatment will cause side effects that interfere with their remaining quality of life, especially when the treatment may extend their life only minimally.

Discussing mortality and death – Even many doctors have difficulty discussing death, and they may use unclear language or avoid the words "death" and "dying." These doctors must be self-aware of their shortcomings and assign this discussion to a nurse, social worker, chaplain, or other appropriate professional. It takes time and skill to discuss mortality.

When the patient has little time to live, the importance of end-of-life plans and advance directives[3] must be discussed. These services can provide meaningful and comforting support to the patient and family regardless of proximity to death. Doctors can also help

---

2   Palliative care is treatment given for the purpose of symptom relief, and it can be used at any time, for any patient, in any situation—it is not only used in the case of terminal illness. Palliative care is often confused with end-of-life care, such as hospice. Hospice provides palliative care at end-of-life, while palliative care can be used during treatment of many non-terminal conditions. Recently, the term "supportive care" is being used in place of "palliative care" for non-terminal patients.

3   Advance directives should always be prepared with the help of medical social workers or other appropriate legal professionals. Refer to the Cancer Harbors module, "Quality of Life," at https://cancerharbors.com/table-of-contents-cancer-harbors/.

patients understand the valuable services hospice provides, such as counseling and support for families and patients.

Physicians should discuss the range and degree of treatment with their patients, remembering that at times, less is more. Minimal treatment may be the best option for comfort at the end of life, enabling a better quality of life for the patient and his or her family. Patients need to be given this option directly and clearly.

Follow-through

Referring to needed services, especially non-medical ones – Doctors are busy and creatures of habit; they often prescribe medication before referring a patient to mental health services, physical therapy, or home health, even when these services are covered by insurance.

Exercise is an important intervention that nearly all patients need. Even when oncologists talk to their patients about exercise, they do not often talk about specific ways to become more active. Patients are likely to listen to their doctor and use the resources the doctor recommends, however (Smaradottir, Smith, Borgert, & Oettel, 2017).

Post-treatment care – Follow-up care, when performed with the patient's quality of life and needs—both anticipated and unanticipated—in mind, can facilitate the healing process and return the patient to function. The underlying causes of dysfunction and disability may go unnoticed during brief follow-up appointments, however. Doctors may not see the manifestations of overtreatment or iatrogenic harm, and consequently they may not refer the patient for rehab or other services unless the patient requests it.

To illustrate, a patient with a gastrointestinal cancer whose small intestine was partly removed may experience difficulty absorbing nutrients following surgery. During this time, he may slowly endure weight loss, chronic diarrhea, and painful skin breakdown. If the patient is not warned of the likelihood of these events, he may not seek professional support, such as nutritional counseling, physical therapy, and behavior modification, which can prevent these conditions from becoming dangerous.

Qualities of Good Care

I emphasize four important qualities of good cancer care: creativity, authenticity, resourceful-ness, and empathy. When cultivated, these contribute to better relationships between patients and physicians and amend the current shortcomings in cancer care.

Creativity

Cookie-cutter approaches to treatment are efficient, but they take creativity and individuality out of the picture. Overworked doctors rely on time-saving measures out of necessity, but real-life issues for patients require creative and critical thought. Breaking out of rigid, linear thinking is necessary and should include interdisciplinary collaboration among many professionals, includ-ing non-medical specialists and community providers.

Community providers and specialists can take the form of cancer coaches who specialize in nutrition, exercise, behavior modification, or health education, or cancer exercise trainers certi-fied by the American Cancer Society or the American College of Sports Medicine, for example.

Many patients would benefit immensely from exercise instruction. They can learn what exercis-es will be most effective, which activities are safe and which should be avoided, and how hard to push themselves. For a patient at risk for lymphedema (swelling in the limbs or other parts of the body), this knowledge can be critical.

Doctors should encourage exercise to reduce the risk of cancer recurrence and promote self-care after treatment. They do not have the time or skill sets to help patients embark on behavior change and lifestyle adjustments, however, so guiding patients to appropriate and needed support through referrals to community providers is a necessary step to improving survivorship care.

Authenticity

Doctors are often pressured to maintain a controlled demeanor, limiting their opportunities for authentic engagement with patients. Hiding behind a façade of stoicism in the face of discomfort, constantly blocking emotions and subjective input, requires doctors to deny their true feelings. This burden leads to separation from their community and being perceived as unapproachable.

It must become more acceptable for doctors to show patients and peers that they engage in self-care and value their own health. Further, they should not feel they must have all the answers. To say, "That is not my scope, but here is someone who can do that for you," is an authentic and creative approach to treatment, instilling trust from patients and the community.

Honesty and forthrightness about treatment limitations and side effects build confidence and trust as well. Fewer people might pursue dangerous or unproven alternatives if doctors would clearly discuss with patients, *up front,* possible negative outcomes of their cancer treatment, such as permanent disability, chronic pain or dysfunction, or lowered quality of life.

Resourcefulness

Resourcefulness is the ability to solve problems by doing the best you can with what you have. Patients' resources are their existing state of health, knowledge, literacy, ability to pay, time, physical and emotional resilience, and support systems. The physician's resources are knowledge and skill in practicing medicine, degree of autonomy and level of support in practice, time available relative to patient load, burden of regulations and insurance-related matters, and satisfaction and enjoyment of their work.

Patients can be resourceful by honing their awareness of the doctor's time and the limitations of the doctor's scope of practice—realizing that the doctor specializes in medicine, not psychosocial or support services. Patients should be prepared to succinctly address their problems with their doctor and request referrals to helpful services. (See the self-advocacy modules of Cancer Harbors at https://cancerharbors.com/table-of-contents-cancer-harbors/.)

Physicians can be resourceful by designating a professional staff member, such as a nurse or social worker, to counsel patients and provide a vetted and up-to-date resource list. This resource list should suggest community resources and service providers, including those outside of the physicians' employers' offerings.

Empathy

Anticipating patients' needs and showing concerns for their quality of life is empathy. Doctors who have been patients are usually able to empathize well, and doctors who have not been in the patient's situation should realize that they can never fully understand it. Doctors should keep this in mind when presenting the entire range of treatment options, including *not treating*.

At diagnosis, doctors must be especially attuned to the patient's grieving process. Patients grieve their loss of control, the loss of their health, and the loss of their ability to put off thoughts of mortality. This grieving process often prevents patients from absorbing much of the information presented at diagnosis, and oncologists must be aware of this.

Oncologists should discuss post-treatment needs with their patients before beginning care. Patients must understand that there is often a cost to treating cancer, and there may be difficult work ahead to restore their prior level of functioning. Above all, oncologists should not minimize the adverse effects or complications, so patients have the ability to make informed decisions about their treatment options.

Improving the Physician Culture and Cancer Care

Doctors need not be heroes; they must be human. They must acknowledge that they cannot provide everything patients need. Without blaming doctors for this state of affairs, we must keep in mind the entrenched paternalism and objective, data-focused culture in which medicine has existed for so long. Changing culture does not happen without great resistance.

By clearly seeing the burdens on doctors and the humans they are, we can support and encourage them to change physician culture. In turn, they will be better able to address patients' needs through follow-up care and community referrals after treatment.

1. **We must change the medical culture of isolation to a collaborative, team-based, community-oriented approach.**

   Doctors' work schedules must include adequate time outside of patient appointments and paperwork to allow for community and interdisciplinary outreach. This collaborative and community-focused approach is more realistic and less isolating. It might even contribute to better job satisfaction and less burnout among physicians. Further, mutual awareness and respect among members of the treatment team will lead to a more holistic and long-term approach to caring for the cancer patient.

2. **We must eliminate the disincentives to medicine as a career.**

   We need to stop making medical school a military drill exercise and instead foster learning in a safe, human-oriented setting. Medical school should be affordable, and the learning experiences should be interdisciplinary. The structure of the medical school curriculum should allow ample time for working with nurses, physical therapists, mental health providers, and other practitioners to help doctors see how important these services are to patient outcomes.

3. Doctors must readily trust and reach out for help from non-medical practitioners.

Time should be allotted in the physician's schedule for learning about other specialties and modalities available to their patients.

4. Doctors need time to engage with their communities.

Oncologists must be visible, personable, approachable, and authentic to regain the trust of a public who often seeks alternative and sometimes dangerous treatments. Doctors are well-respected and can promote public understanding of science to dispel myths and misinformation.

5. Qualitative research methods used in social and behavioral sciences should be utilized in medical research and practice.

Ignoring psychosocial and quality of life issues because they are subjective leads to dismissal of important patient anecdotes and qualitative measures. Since health is closely tied to behavior, a behavioral approach to research is of utmost importance. The longer we focus only on clinical evidence and ignore first-person anecdotes, the longer we will delay making progress in improving patients' lives around cancer treatment.

6. Patients and physicians must relate to each other on an equal level, as human beings.

The doctor may be the expert on the science and application of cancer treatment, but patients are experts on themselves. There should be mutual communication, collaboration, and respect, and the ability to have a conversation on equal footing once each side is brought up to speed on the other's expertise.

7. Physicians who have not had cancer should be aware that they cannot fully understand patients' and survivors' needs.

Physicians who lack firsthand knowledge of the physical, emotional, sexual, spiritual, and financial needs of cancer survivors should be aware of their shortcomings. They must refer patients to other professionals, so patients may find the best solutions and resources for their needs.

What Can Physicians Do?

Physicians can start by defining their values. A simple Values Exercise (page A8) should be repeated on a regular basis throughout one's medical career. The resulting statement of values can be placed on a website for prospective patients to read.

Physicians should begin by thinking about their personal mission in medicine—why they entered the practice. Thinking forward to what they want to accomplish by the end of their career, they can decide whether the path they are on is taking them there. Do they need to correct their course? Should they turn around, change directions, bail out, or let the ship sink? What is the cost to them if they do not?

Physicians need humane education programs, good social and communication skills, and time to network professionally and engage with their non-medical communities. This will lead to understanding outside a narrow area of specialization, and will allow doctors to acknowledge their humanity. This will go a long way toward better care for cancer patients and happier, more successful doctors.

Calls to Action for Physicians

» Physicians are not heroes, and they shouldn't try to be. They should not be expected to transcend their own humanity. They can exhibit compassion for their patients and for themselves. For the sake of self-preservation, they must take care of their own physical and mental health. Besides, if they were superhuman, how would they relate to their mortal patients?

» Physicians must step out of the shelter of their offices and organizations to interact with their communities and learn how non-medical and complementary service providers can support their patients. Being visible and approachable in the community will earn them trust and credibility.

References

American Medical Association. (2004). *Toward defining paternalism in medicine*. Retrieved March 15, 2017, from http://journalofethics.ama-assn.org/2004/02/fred1-0402.html

Andrew, L. B. (2016). *Physician suicide*. Retrieved March 20, 2017, from http://emedicine.medscape.com/article/806779-overview

Barnlund, D. C. (1970). A transactional model of communication. In Akin, J., Goldberg, A., Myers, G., & Steward, J. (Eds.), *Language behavior: A book of readings in communication* (pp. 43-61). The Hague, Netherlands: Mouton & Co. Publishers.

Brawley, O. W. (2011). *How we do harm: A doctor breaks ranks about being sick in America*. New York: St. Martin's Press.

Cox, A. M. (2016, December 28). *New York Times Magazine*. Retrieved March 20, 2017, from https://www.nytimes.com/2016/12/28/magazine/vivek-murthy-thinks-we-need-to-learn-how-to-deal-with-stress.html?_r=0

Hoffmann, T. C. & Del Mar, C. (2017). Clinicians' expectations of the benefits and harms of treatments, screening, and tests: A systematic review. *JAMA Internal Medicine, 177*(3), 407-419. doi:10.1001/jamainternmed.2016.8254

Kavilanz, P. B. (2009, July 18). *Family doctors: An endangered breed*. Retrieved March 15, 2017, from http://money.cnn.com/2009/07/16/news/economy/healthcare_doctors_shortage/

Lipsenthal, L. (2005). The physician personality: Confronting our perfectionism and social isolation. *Holistic and Primary Care, 6*(3). Retrieved March 19, 2017, from https://holisticprimarycare.net/topics/topics-o-z/reflections/200-the-physician-personality-confronting-our-perfectionism-and-social-isolation.html

Merriam-Webster. (n.d.). *Iatrogenesis*. Retrieved March 19, 2017, from https://www.merriam-webster.com/medical/iatrogenesis

National Academy of Sciences. (2009). *Supply and demand in the oncology workforce*. Retrieved March 15, 2017, from https://www.ncbi.nlm.nih.gov/books/NBK215252/

Pho, K. (2011, June 20). *Why the AMA is in decline, and should doctors care?* Retrieved March

15, 2017, from http://www.kevinmd.com/blog/2011/06/ama-decline-doctors-care.html

Smaradottir, A., Smith, A. L., Borgert, A. J., & Oettel, K. R. (2017). Are we on the same page? Patient and provider perceptions about exercise in cancer care: A focus group study. *Journal of the National Comprehensive Cancer Network, 15*(5), 588-594. doi:10.6004/jnccn.2017.0061

TEDMED. (2016, March 23). Pamela Wible: Why doctors kill themselves [Video file]. Retrieved March 20, 2017, from https://www.youtube.com/watch?v=qyVAtZ9VZ4Q

Chapter Four: Eye of the Storm

Nurses' roles in cancer survivorship care

"Sometimes we just have to create the movement, tribe, teachings, revolution, and evolution that we want to be a part of."

– Annette Tersigni, RN, CEO & Founder of YogaNurse®[1]

Nurses have knowledge, skills, and ability to provide safe passage through the process of cancer treatment. Patients should be informed about nurses' expert roles in health and patient care—and how they differ from physicians'—so they can take advantage of nursing services. After all, nurses spend more time in direct care of patients than any other healthcare worker.

A healthcare system that values nurses and expands their role in cancer care would relieve many problems from prevention through survivorship. In this chapter, I will discuss the importance of nurses, their roles, and their preparation. Then I will discuss how the current healthcare model limits what nurses can bring to cancer care, and I will propose solutions to expand nursing roles to benefit cancer patients and educate the public about cancer.

What Is a Nurse?

The public often does not understand all of what nurses do and the importance of their work. Doctors receive the most attention, but nurses, social workers, dietitians, and physical, occupational, and speech therapists do important footwork. These healthcare professionals safely take a patient from diagnosis through treatment, teaching and guiding them to healing and comfort.

Nurses play key roles in helping the patient survive. The doctor plans the treatment, while nurses ensure the treatment is carried out safely and effectively. They address adverse

---

1   Tersigni, n.d.

treatment effects that might endanger the patient's life or well-being. They provide information, resources, and support along the way.

Nurses are educated in anatomy, physiology, and pathological processes of disease. They are well-versed in pharmacology, understanding the actions of drugs, side effects, dosage, and more. Nurses administer drugs and watch the patient for reactions.

Nurses perform physical assessments, document their findings in the chart, and report abnormalities to the physician. Nurses teach patients about the drugs they are taking and what to do after surgery. They stop a procedure from happening if the chart says one thing and the doctor says another. Their tasks are as varied as listening to a patient's lungs, making sure medical equipment is working properly, and watching for signs of malnutrition, abuse, or lack of support at home.

During a bedside procedure, nurses administer sedation, check that the patient's heart rhythm is normal, and monitor breathing. Because of the intense focus on the procedure, the doctor may not know if the patient's heart went into a dangerous rhythm, if he is over-sedated, or that he needs more oxygen. Nurses watch for these signs of distress, however, and they act on them.

Nurses relate to patients on a human level, relieving suffering, providing comfort, and meeting their functional and practical needs. They watch for subtle changes in the patient's condition. Nurses know about nutrition, functional activities of daily living, and resources to help their patients with physical, emotional, social, occupational, and spiritual needs. They educate patients in self-care and proper use of medications.

Nurses watch patients twenty-four hours a day; they are the safety check. They are the eyes, ears, nose, voice, feet, and hands of healthcare. They are responsible for all these duties, and they are doing them on several patients at the same time.

Other Healthcare Professionals

Patients interact with many other medical professionals, such as navigators, social workers, and case managers, during their cancer care. It can be helpful to understand their various roles and responsibilities, as well as their limitations. For example, medical assistants are trained in administrative and clinical tasks. If a patient reports a concerning symptom to a medical assistant, he or she may not be able to discern whether it is a minor concern or a life-threatening emergency. A nurse, on the other hand, would know how to respond.

(The self-advocacy section of the appendix, page A39, provides an explanation of medical staff who work closely with nurses and physicians.)

Training for Oncology Nurses

The basic requirement for an oncology nurse is the RN (registered nurse) license, which presently requires, at minimum, an Associate's Degree in Nursing (ADN). (Some hospitals now require a Bachelor of Science in Nursing.) Nurses take courses in pharmacology, microbiology, anatomy and physiology, human development, psychology, chemistry, ethics, pathophysiology, nutrition, and statistics, even at the Associate's degree level.

After a nurse has a license and is practicing, continuing education requirements vary by state. Nurses may join professional organizations for their specific area of practice: critical care, oncology, orthopedics, and many others. Nurses can obtain certifications for specialized areas of nursing. The Certified Oncology Nurse (OCN) is the basic certification for RNs in oncology, and the Oncology Nursing Society is the leading professional organization for oncology nurses.

In oncology, Advanced Practice Nurses (APRNs or NPs)—nurses who are at least Master's level trained and usually able to prescribe drugs and perform certain interventions not within the scope of RNs—often prescribe medications for symptom relief, screen for recurrence, educate, provide survivorship follow-up care, and manage patient care at a more advanced level during treatment (Wainstock & Sevedge, 1998).

Tasks of Oncology Nurses

Oncology nurses are responsible for ensuring patients receive treatments or drugs safely and correctly and that symptoms are managed to provide comfort. Doctors' orders are carefully confirmed, labs are drawn, and the patient's physical condition is confirmed to be adequate for a dose of chemotherapy. All medications must be double-checked with another nurse or the pharmacist and rechecked at the patient's side. These measures take time and concentration.

Special training is required for nurses who administer chemotherapy drugs, for safety reasons. Chemotherapy chemicals are extremely toxic; protective clothing and equipment must be worn and precautions must be taken to avoid chemotherapy spills.

The Culture of Nursing and Its Impact on Patient Care

Modern nursing began in the 19th century. While nurses' responsibilities, duties, and education have changed dramatically, the paternalistic and self-sacrificial ways have stuck through modern times.

Nurses have high rates of job turnover. Like physicians, the cumulative and repetitive traumas of the job make nurses vulnerable to stress-induced physical and mental illness. PTSD is common (Mealer et al, 2009), but some nurses avoid treatment because nursing boards inquire about mental health on licensing applications and renewals. Nurses who admit to depression or other mental illness may have to justify their fitness to work.

Nurses and physicians have much in common, in their approach to work, their professional culture, their self-neglect, and the effect their behavior has on patient care. Both simply try to make it through each task-filled day and collapse at the end of the shift, functioning within their own silos. Thus, there is no mutual acknowledgement of the sense of community or shared purpose among the healthcare team.

Nurses are educated holistically but become exhausted and overwhelmed by their countless specialized tasks. They are not allotted time for further holistic, community-oriented training to improve patient outcomes and survivorship. For example, many oncology nurses would benefit from further education on metastatic cancer, as well as meeting patients' psychosocial needs after treatment.

When nurses do receive continuing education or attend professional conferences, many programs are sponsored by drug companies, which pay for nurses' dinners while they market the latest infusion drug. This limits the opportunities to learn about non-pharmaceutical advances in patient care.

Nurses report feeling unsupported and undervalued by management (Johnston et al., 2016), and feel their jobs may be at risk if they speak up for safety concerns (Agency for Healthcare Research and Quality, 2016; Okuyama, Wagner, & Bijnen, 2014). The dangers of for-profit interests to healthcare and patient safety have been identified (Brock & Buchanan, 1986), but nurses' concerns often take a back seat to profit in the healthcare industry's business approach.

The Magnet[2] designation, for example, is used as a public relations tool (DeTora, n.d.; Packer, 2017), but organizations often find work-arounds to improve their fiscal results at the expense of nurses' job satisfaction and patient safety (Summers, 2016).

Nurses must understand that they are not working in the best interest of their patients when they are martyrs to their work. An atmosphere of coercion and fear is not conducive to patient advocacy.

Nurses and physicians could make a powerful statement as a team. Together, they can stand up to management with strong, organized self-representation.

Improving Nursing Culture and Cancer Care

Nursing and healthcare cultures and their dysfunctions affect cancer care and survivorship. Nurses can do better by clarifying the importance of their roles. It's important for the public and all stakeholders in healthcare to understand what nurses can and should be doing to benefit cancer survivors.

Nurses need to lead this effort by acting forcefully and demanding change. Advocacy is needed, and nurses need to be courageous—not martyrs—and remember their duty to patient safety. Nurses must consider important issues, such as how their day-to-day efforts are making in difference in quality of life for patients during and after treatment.

In my experience in the hospital setting, I felt patients needed much more than just chemotherapy infusions. Nurses should be utilized after treatment as educators, survivorship coaches, and navigators. With their holistic approach, nurses are the ideal experts to offer these services. Long-term costs associated with poor health could be reduced, and quality of life may be enhanced for survivors. Presently, this is not covered by insurance, however. Further, healthcare management should view nurses by the value they add to the patient experience and to the greater well-being of society.

I want everyone to understand how important well-functioning nurses are to safe and effective cancer survivorship care, for patients, their family members, and other stakeholders in healthcare. Once again, creativity, authenticity, resourcefulness, and empathy are key qualities of care.

---

2   Magnet is a credentialing designation given to hospitals that is supposed to measure the quality of nursing services in a facility. The facility must meet certain performance criteria in nursing workplace standards and in providing nursing care to patients.

Nurses and patients can benefit from the following points on an improved nursing approach.

1. **Nurses must heal themselves if they are to heal others.**

   Nursing culture needs to change. Nurses cannot help people heal when they work in toxic settings. Nurses must stop the epidemic of dysfunction and abuse within the profession and take responsibility for acting as professionals.

2. **Health, well-being, and quality of life are important, and self-care is necessary to achieve these ideals.**

   Nurses need to take better physical and emotional care of themselves. They need support, debriefing after traumatic events, physical exercise, and good nutritional practices. They need empathy for themselves and their colleagues and to be authentically themselves.

3. **Nurses must demand additional resources for nursing care.**

   Nurses need administrators and executives to support them in fulfilling their duties. Nurses need additional support staff for patient care, as well as staff coverage to take breaks. Nurses should be allowed to use their education and critical thinking skills in caring for individual patient needs, rather than working on autopilot for 12 or 13 hours at a stretch. Nurses will not get the respect they deserve until they demand it.

4. **Healthcare providers should witness individual, community, and public health realities and how they affect people's lives.**

   Nurses should be visible in the community—in schools, public forums, and senior centers, for example, teaching about health, disease prevention, and medications. They are trained to provide this education but rarely have time to do it. Nurses can act as health coaches, influencing everyday behavior in long-term maintenance of health.

5. **Oncology care and greater healthcare should adopt a team approach—an interdisciplinary, mutually respectful process that fully includes nurses in the healthcare team.**

   All caregivers must allocate time in their schedules to meet as teams. Nurses, doctors, navigators, social workers, dietitians, mental health workers, and physical, occupational, and speech therapists should come together regularly to discuss a patient's care. Rather than focusing solely on the medical treatment, other aspects of care can be attended to early on. A team approach allows for planning and treatment with survivorship in mind.

6. Nursing education must change.

Nurses and physicians should be trained alongside each other during parts of their education to foster mutual understanding, respect, trust, autonomy, and division of labor. During nursing school, nurses should be exposed to employment alternatives outside of hospitals to gain a broader perspective of healthcare. Nurse training should be less task-focused and more overarching, looking at the bigger picture of the patient's life before and after cancer treatment.

7. Wining and dining by drug companies should be removed from oncology continuing education.

Too many lightweight, passive dinner meetings are sponsored by drug company representatives, where nurses absorb little more than a glass of wine. Instead, continuing education should inform nurses about the broader scope of nursing in the community and long-term patient outcomes.

8. Nurses should not be discouraged from using social media.

Many nurses are afraid to use social media because their employers threaten them with termination for potentially breaching patient privacy. But social media can be used in a way that does not breach patient privacy. Social media can allow nurses to interact with their peers all over the country and the world, to share ideas, support each other, and see how other nurses boost their enjoyment of work and improve patient care. On Twitter, for example, oncology nurses can participate in interdisciplinary chats with patients and other oncology professionals.

9. Professional nursing organizations must act in the best interest of nurses.

They must encourage outspokenness and self-advocacy by nurses working in direct patient care, embrace entrepreneurship among nurses, showcase opportunities for non-academic and non-traditional nursing endeavors, and avoid drug company domination of professional conference and educational offerings. They thus will ensure that patient safety and nurses' ability to provide the highest quality care will be prioritized at all times.

Alternatives to Traditional Nursing Employment

After leaving traditional healthcare, I was fortunate to find Nurseup.com. Founded by Andrew Lopez, RN, it is a group of nurse entrepreneurs who support each other, collaborate, network, and share their expertise as true professional colleagues.

Healthy Nurse by Design (http://lisbethoverton.com), founded by Lisbeth Overton, RN, started as an online organization to support nurses and build trust and camaraderie among nursing professionals. It has now evolved to promote wellness and self-care for all women. Workshop participants learn skills in emotional and physical self-nurturing for coping with stress, and they experience personal and spiritual growth. Her own experiences with stress-related illness inspired her to help other women overcome the culture of self-neglect and to redefine their purpose and value.

These nurses are my peers now: creative, authentic, resourceful, and empathetic. We see problems and figure out ways to solve them. The common thread uniting us all is our desire to improve healthcare for nurses, patients, and the greater public. It is a grassroots effort far removed from the bloated bureaucracies of big healthcare. When one of us succeeds, we bring others up with us.

I look forward to a day when people no longer dramatize my work as an oncology nurse.

"You must be an angel!"

"That must be so depressing."

"How can you do that? It must be so hard."

"God bless you, I could never…."

I cannot count the number of times I have heard these statements, even from other nurses! Healthcare professionals must stop seeing cancer from the antiquated view that equates it with a death sentence. They must also stop making the assumption that death is to be avoided at all costs.

I have not found oncology to be depressing. Oncology nursing is an opportunity to make a difference in outcomes as well as prevention. I have seen people face their greatest fears and come out the other side with strength and confidence they never knew they had, or to accept the end of their lives with grace and peace. I have lost patients, clients, and friends over the years to cancer, but I have learned that taking the time to acknowledge my feelings and honor my grief keeps me grounded. Death is a part of life, and nurses see it every day. Living your life fully is the greatest gift you can give yourself.

I want to educate people about cancer so they can face it and see it for what it is: a different situation in every instance. I want patients to have the skills to create the best outcome and quality of life for themselves, regardless of life expectancy, prognosis for their cancer, and their treatment plan.

It is great and honorable to be an oncology nurse, but nurses need options. Then nursing work will be a conscious choice, and perhaps nurses will be more likely to make needed changes to their profession. The mainstream workplace burned me out, but I found a way to relight my candle. I can only hope that I can relight other extinguished candles along the way.

Nurses must be visible, acknowledged, appreciated, and valued, and they also must fully understand their value and articulate it. They must remember that doing no harm means speaking out and advocating for patient safety. They must respect themselves as professionals and whole human beings who are worthy of work environments in which their physical and mental well-being are respected. That will be the first of many difficult steps toward making their working conditions better, and in the end, improving cancer survivorship.

Calls to Action for Nurses

» Nurses must take responsibility for pulling the expectations of their profession out of the dark ages. They cannot be afraid to advocate for themselves and for their patients by demanding more staff and an end to the exploitative labor practices of the healthcare industry. Furthermore, they should not be expected to sacrifice their own safety or physical and mental well-being to do their jobs. This, in turn, will result in better, more attentive patient care.

» Nurses should insist that their education builds pride in professionalism and shows student nurses a broad range of opportunities. They must keep their intellectual curiosity alive by engaging in opportunities to learn, unobstructed by the limited offerings that result from reliance on industry funding.

References

Agency for Healthcare Research and Quality. (2016). Hospital survey on patient safety culture: 2016 user comparative database report. Retrieved October 20, 2017, from www.ahrq.gov/sites/default/files/wysiwyg/professionals/quality-patient-safety/patientsafetyculture/hospital/2016/2016_hospitalsops_report_pt1.pdf

Brock, D. W. & Buchanan, A. (1986). Ethical issues in for-profit health care. In B. H. Gray (Ed.), *Institute of Medicine (U.S.) Committee on Implications of For-Profit Enterprise in Health Care*. Washington, D.C.: National Academies Press. Retrieved October 20, 2017, from https://www.ncbi.nlm.nih.gov/books/NBK217902/

DeTora, G. (n.d.) Magnet designation can be a powerful branding tool. Retrieved October 20, 2017, from http://www.detoraconsulting.com/published-articles/magnet-designation-can-be-a-powerful-branding-tool-2

Johnston, D., Bell, C., Jones, M., Farquharson, B., Allan, J., Schofield, P., et al. (2016). Stressors, appraisal of stressors, experienced stress and cardiac response: A real-time, real-life investigation of work stress in nurses. *Annals of Behavioral Medicine, 50*(2), 187-197. doi:10.1007/s12160-015-9746-8

Mealer, M., Burnham, E. L., Goode, C. J., Rothbaum, B. and Moss, M. (2009). The prevalence and impact of post traumatic stress disorder and burnout syndrome in nurses. *Depression and Anxiety, 26*(12), 1118-1126. doi:10.1002/da.20631

Okuyama, A., Wagner, C., & Bijnen, B. (2014). Speaking up for patient safety by hospital-based health care professionals: A literature review. *BMC Health Services Research, 14*, 61. doi:10.1186/1472-6963-14-61

Packer, M. (2017, September 27). Do hospitals get prestigious national awards for poor nursing? *MedPage Today*. Retrieved October 20, 2017, from https://www.medpagetoday.com/Blogs/RevolutionandRevelation/68162

Summers, S. (2016, October 2). Magnet status: What it is, what it is not, and what it could be. Retrieved October 20, 2017, from http://www.truthaboutnursing.org/faq/magnet.html

Tersigni, A. [Annette]. (n.d.) Sometimes we just have to create the movement...[Pinterest post]. Retrieved November 20, 2017, from https://www.pinterest.com/pin/85849936628002136/

Wainstock, J. M. & Sevedge, K. (1998). Roles of advanced practice nurses in oncology. *Cancer Network*, *12*(4). Retrieved March 30, 2017, from http://www.cancernetwork.com/review-article/ roles-advanced-practice-nurses-oncology

Chapter Five: Captains and Pirates on the High Seas

Healthcare administrators, leaders, and decision-makers

"Not everything that can be counted counts. Not everything that counts can be counted."

– Sociologist William Bruce Cameron[1]

Healthcare is a human service, with good health, well-being, and quality of life as the ideal outcomes. It should be considered in a qualitative light, in terms of patients' results and public health outcomes. Healthcare jargon talks about "delivery" of the product "healthcare," but it cannot be run like a factory; we are not producing a product. People involved in healthcare administration and policymaking say they are delivering "value," but they would do well to understand what this means for the quality of a patient's life.

The focus of this chapter is how the actions of healthcare administrators, executives, policymakers, and legislators impact cancer survivorship, as I have experienced as a nurse "down here." My intent is not to rant and rave against a system at which I sometimes feel overwhelmed and powerless, but to call attention to matters that are unresolved.

I must first stress that there are many good people doing good work in healthcare. There are great leaders who exemplify honesty, transparency, and respect for the people who work for them and the people they serve. There are leaders who strive to serve both the direct caregivers—doctors, nurses, and other healthcare workers they employ—and the end-users of the services they oversee—that is, the patients and their families. Serve is a key word here. When leaders seek to serve, all ships rise.

---

1   Cameron, 1967, p. 13

But too often, from my viewpoint as a nurse, those in elected and leadership positions do not address issues such as patient outcomes and healthcare workers' ability to provide safe patient care—not with true understanding and empathy for their concerns. These issues are raised repeatedly, but impactful changes that favor patients' needs over profit are rarely implemented.

I believe deeply that businesspeople, elected officials, and policymakers, as well as those who influence them, must acknowledge their part in creating an opportunistic healthcare culture that is set up for profit over patient care. While executives and leaders in healthcare are doing the fiscally-driven work they know how to do, their work has great impact on healthcare professionals' ability to care for patients—patients who may be hanging on to hope that they will survive and see better days.

The proliferation of social media groups among nurses and other healthcare workers, and the discussions taking place there, provide evidence that many healthcare workers hold these viewpoints and desire to bring these issues to national attention. My views are widely shared with other nurses, and they are not localized to any one healthcare system or region of the country.

In this chapter, I discuss the character of the healthcare industry regarding direct patient care, which sets the stage for understanding the impact on cancer patient outcomes. I include anecdotes from nurses in hospitals across the country to illustrate my points.

Relationships Between Executives/Administrators and Direct Patient Care Staff

There is a two-tiered system of professionals in healthcare: the providers—those who directly care for patients, such as nurses, doctors, and other clinical specialists—and the "suits"—those who oversee the daily operations of healthcare facilities, such as managers, administrators, and executives.

There is little discussion between the two regarding purpose, planning, and needs. From the standpoint of providers, it often seems that upper management is unaccountable to patients or their clinical caregivers. Instead, direct care providers may perceive micromanagement, with an abundance of expectations, regulations, and requirements from both inside and outside the organization. Executives make decisions behind closed doors, and the decisions are revealed only when they are announced to staff. These decisions may add to the clinical workload, and staff scramble to make sense of changes in the context of their own aims for patient care: safety and favorable outcomes.

Many executives were trained in business or healthcare administration. Of those who have patient care experience, many are long removed from direct care. (Middle managers are more likely to have direct experience in the departments they manage.)

Speaking Different Languages

Executive jargon abounds in healthcare administration—*customers* instead of *patients*, *products delivered* instead of *care given*, *staff* instead of *professionals* or *clinicians*, *providers* instead of *doctors* or *nurses*. This alternate language provides administrators an opaque shield that hinders outside understanding.

Moreover, feel-good buzzwords are thrown around, but results often do not match the implied benefits of these words. Let's look at a few and discuss what they mean for cancer survivorship.

The phrase "patient-centered care" has been around for some time and describes a variety of changes that accommodate patient needs—from more permissive visiting hours and higher quality hospital food, to more clinically-oriented changes in direct care. In cancer care, the American Society for Clinical Oncology (ASCO) policy statement on "patient-centered health-care reform" specifies principles to ensure high quality cancer care (ASCO, 2017).

Notably missing in the ASCO statement, however, are direct references to optimal quality of life and comfort, palliative care services, and post-treatment or survivorship care services. The statement contains the phrase "full range of services," but the full range of patient needs are not specified.

The new Oncology Care Model by the Center for Medicare and Medicaid Services (2016) has been implemented to control costs of cancer care by compensating physicians for value-based care instead of fee-for-service. Workloads and caseloads remain high, however. There are still barriers to accessing care and still high stress among care providers. The public is still not sufficiently educated on the importance of preventive health strategies and does not know about valuable services such as navigation and mental health care. These significant problems must be overcome to make progress in improving oncology care. Mere mentions of "patient-centered care" will not be enough until organizations commit to making changes work in the system, such as offering mental health services to patients—and sufficiently staffing for them.

Another healthcare buzzword is "engagement." Healthcare administrators use it to describe the relative level of cooperation and attitude of clinical staff. Engagement is presumed low when frustration and burnout among doctors and nurses is high. A cottage industry of consulting services attempts to improve provider engagement.

Poor engagement in doctors and nurses can result from a lack of transparency and communication, as well as homogeneity in viewpoints on the part of administrators. A lack of participation in administrative meetings by clinical staff contributes as well. Most hospital boards are dominated by business executives (and may include physicians with business degrees). Few nurses are included in influential positions on hospital boards. Actively practicing nurses are almost never present for boardroom discussions.

Consequences of Communication Gaps

Most hospitals are now part of large healthcare corporations; the bigger the organization, the more bureaucratic the decision-making process becomes. Frequently, decisions affecting care staff are made in remote offices by people who have never worked as direct care providers. High-tech, expensive, or complicated solutions are implemented from afar, even when decision-makers have little idea of the impact on the ground. Consequently, care staff often show considerable resentment, anger, and resistance to changes brought about by executives when they perceive the changes to be detrimental to patient care.

Anecdote: The trash cans

A high-level administrator observed the patient rooms in his hospital. The trash cans, he noted, were not aesthetically pleasing. The dull, gray, columnar cans with open tops and visible plastic liners looked distasteful to him. He decided stainless steel, lidded trash cans would make the room look more sanitary.

What the administrator did not realize was that nurses frequently toss waste items toward the open trash cans, saving time by disposing of waste without contaminating their hands. Time is the scarcest resource in a nurse's day; even trash cans with foot pedals require nurses to walk back and forth across the room, requiring more time to complete basic tasks. If the lid sticks, their hands become contaminated, and they must de-glove, wash their hands, and re-glove.

Without having consulted nursing staff, the administrator ordered 300 lidded trash cans. After they were placed in the patient rooms, the nurses were up in arms. Simple tasks, such as flushing IVs or taking temperatures, which nurses may perform multiple times per shift on multiple patients, suddenly required considerable extra effort, as nurses had to cross the room to dispose of syringes or thermometer covers.

If the administrator had consulted the nurses, they could have chosen a trash can that satisfied both aesthetics and practicality. At $200 per trash can, this $60,000 mistake could have been avoided.

Perceptions of Administration by Clinical Staff

Accurate or not, hospital staff commonly possess certain perceptions of executives. These typically include:

1. They benefit from a culture of entitlement.

Executives hold retreats at expensive resort communities, stay at nice hotels, and eat at nice restaurants. They play golf, travel in first class, and have catered meetings, special parking spots, and luxurious offices behind locked and secured entrances. They live in nice homes and take extravagant vacations. Their secretaries answer their emails and phones, and they can avoid directly answering to anyone they do not wish to hear from.

2. They are sheltered from the day-to-day realities of healthcare.

Administrators are seldom seen on the hospital floor except when surrounded by other people in suits. Many clinical staff only ever glimpse administrators when they are reading the local newspaper—pictured at the groundbreaking of a new facility (always appearing in a suit under a hardhat), and later at the ribbon cutting for that new facility (always in a suit with a pair of scissors).

Anecdote: Death on Christmas Day

When I worked in the ICU, I always worked on Christmas. Each year it seemed I had a patient who was dying. One Christmas, I was caring for a patient who was within hours of death. Her family members were in and out of the room, paying their last respects. The room's privacy curtain was partially drawn, but with the traffic in and out it didn't stay closed.

I was just outside the room when two figures approached in the hallway. Dressed in jeans and sweaters, I did not recognize them at first, but quickly realized they were the hospital's

Chief Nursing Officer and Chief Financial Officer. They were thanking staff for working on Christmas. They made casual conversation with me for a few minutes, until a family member stepped out of the patient's room, casting the curtain aside just enough for the executives to see in.

My patient was pale but peaceful, propped up on pillows with smooth sheets pulled up to her chest, her mouth slightly open and eyes closed. She was unresponsive, looking as close to death as anyone could, but her heart was still beating. I heard an audible gasp from one of the executives. He had not realized before that moment what my assignment was behind the curtain. When they stepped away after a little more conversation, they thanked me profusely and sincerely.

I have not forgotten that day and their reaction because I have not experienced anything like it again. On Christmas Day in the ICU, I was caring for a dying woman and her family—for me, a typical day, but not something they thought much about in their work. The world of the executives was so detached from ours that they were genuinely startled to see death in front of them.

3. They receive excessive compensation.

Executives receive far greater compensation than anyone who works directly with patients. In addition to their high salaries, they receive numerous benefits and perks, earn bonuses based on growth or profit margins, and, if they lose their job—even for incompetence—they are entitled to compensation that can be equal to the lifetime earnings of a clinical staff member.

4. They do not always actively listen.

Executives make decisions based on the bottom line and are distracted from the well-being of patients. They rarely or inconsistently gather feedback from employees to improve care.

Anecdote: The *C. Diff* Outbreak

A hospital inpatient oncology unit was experiencing a high rate of *C. diff* transmission among patients on the floor. *C. diff* is healthcare lingo for *Clostridium difficile*, a type of bacteria that is highly contagious and is transmitted in hospitals and the community. It is traced to overuse of antibiotics.

The inpatient oncology unit used to experience occasional *C. diff* infections, but the frequency of the outbreaks had been increasing steadily in recent months. The hospital had recently invested in high-tech equipment for sanitizing the rooms between patients, and it had tightened its monitoring of the use of personal protective equipment (such as gowns, gloves, and masks) for contact isolation rooms. It also provided numerous reminders to care staff about handwashing and alcohol hand gel use between patients. The hospital had also discussed overuse of antibiotics with physicians to attempt to control the conditions that contribute to *C. diff*.

The administration also chose to monitor everyone's hand hygiene practices and even installed cameras to keep a closer watch. Nurses blamed other staff for being noncompliant with hand hygiene, but upon monitoring, it was found that all were compliant with the policy of using either alcohol hand gel or handwashing.

The *C. diff* problem persisted, however, because evidence shows that alcohol does not kill *C. diff*. The best way to control it is vigorous, old-fashioned handwashing.

The staff, therefore, needed to be educated that alcohol gel does not kill *C. diff*. They needed to comply with handwashing, not gel use. Handwashing takes time, so more staff were also needed, so they would not be so rushed.

The administration thought technology in the form of sanitizing equipment would fix the problem. What they needed, however, was basic: more staff and more education. They needed to understand that patient care entails taking the time to do basic tasks that keep patients safe.

Executives needed to see for themselves how the problem manifested on the floor. Because they did not examine the true problem, however, they wasted money on unneeded equipment and created an unpleasant environment for the staff who were being monitored.

5. **They are not accountable to direct patient care staff, patients, and the community.**

If the administration is not accountable directly to patients and employees, to whom are they held accountable? In a for-profit organization, they are accountable to the shareholders; in a not-for-profit organization, it is to their board. Accountability to the staff and to the patients is not a priority.

How Administrative Actions Affect Cancer Patients and Survivorship

The focus on business operations, profitability, competition, and data collection can be at odds with providing services and care during human beings' weakest and most vulnerable moments. Providing high quality patient care can be difficult for healthcare workers when administrators' expectations, in service of their business goals, undercut care staff's abilities to live up to their professional, scientific, moral, and ethical obligations.

1. Mission vs. action

Healthcare organizations write lofty, altruistic-sounding mission statements to say they care about patients and communities. They use clichéd phrases such as, "all under one roof," "we make lives better," "personalized care," "game changers," and "world-class care."

Capital expenses like new radiation machines and surgical robotics, some of which have not been proven superior over older, less expensive versions, allow a hospital bragging rights in a competitive industry. And when every healthcare center has similar facilities and treatment options, they find other ways to attract customers: highway billboards advertising short ER waiting times, or community health fairs and screening events to diagnose people with prostate cancer so the radiation and robotic machines can be paid for. Expensive and high-tech machines do not equate to good care, however.

2. Ethics

The American College of Healthcare Executives displays its ethics statement on its website (ACHE Commitment to Ethics, n.d.). Administrators who were truly bound to these ethical standards would acknowledge the realistic value they add to patient and public health outcomes, and eliminate their own jobs, not clinical staff! Administrative expenditures have grown exponentially compared to spending on clinical staff (Adamopoulos, 2014), while public health outcomes in the U.S. are worse than in other industrialized nations and we have more chronic health conditions and associated costs.

We must improve the worth of healthcare by removing anything that does not add value: insurance company requirements, the time providers and patients spend on authorizations and claim denials, ridiculous prices for drugs, reliance on technology even when it does not create better outcomes, regulations that create more paperwork without demonstrated benefit, and administrative costs of running facilities that are staffed with high-paid paper pushers who make more work for the direct care providers.

3. Data collection for the sake of itself

Is no one is tracking the benefits or detriments of collecting massive amounts of healthcare data known as "metrics?" Accountability should be to improved quality of life, as defined by cancer patients. Are patients receiving adequate and safe care to restore their health or keep them comfortable?

4. Fiscal responsibility

Measures to reduce waste in healthcare could save billions of dollars annually (Mirza, 2017). With the merging of healthcare systems and the trend of building new cancer centers come additional expenses. For example, each time a healthcare facility joins a different entity, its logo changes. The cost of changing everything—printed materials, signs, uniforms, the list is endless—uses financial resources that could be allocated to actual care of patients.

5. PR and marketing

In the fiercely competitive market for healthcare, each organization tries to show it has an edge on competing facilities. They advertise their technologically advanced services, the shortest waiting times, better outcomes, or amenities that other organizations cannot boast. Full-page color advertisements appear in local newspapers, and billboards are placed prominently throughout communities. In cancer care, some of the more egregious claims of better outcomes or survival rates have been revealed as false advertising that preys on the desperation of patients and families (Begley & Respaut, 2013). The sizable budgets dedicated to marketing and public relations in these organizations show that getting good press is a priority.

Awards are another way for hospitals to claim an edge on their competition. Many of these awards are not actually "won;" they come down to jumping through hoops to meet criteria and paying some amount of money to receive certain awards. (How the hospital pays is not always clear; sometimes the awarding organization performs consulting work for the hospital, for example. The point is, it is not exactly a level playing field.)

Top 100 awards are used routinely by hospitals in advertising, but the Top 100 use only certain quality ratings or measurements as criteria (Rau, 2013). These ratings and measurements may not be representative of the quality of patient outcomes.

Hospitals and cancer centers should instead reveal to the public their safety-related measures of quality: hospital-acquired infections, readmissions, errors, violations discovered in inspections by government agencies, fines, and lawsuits. Specific to cancer, consumers should know how many chemotherapy errors there have been, how many navigators are available for patients, the range of treatment services available, and the availability and quality of follow-up or post-treatment services.

6. Staffing

Human bodies and minds do not function like a factory; they can't suddenly pick up their pace and crank more patients through the system. They can function for only so long before they need rest. Humans only heal at a certain rate, but this principle seems to be lost on production-and-efficiency-minded administrators. Asking staff to work harder and with more patients at the same rate of healing is a losing battle.

Further, cutting direct care staff to reduce costs is not aligned with patients' healing. Nurses are an expense, and policies that cut nursing staff create unsafe conditions for patients. Nurses cannot be made to rush through chemotherapy administration, to shorten the time they spend with patients recovering from sedation, or to administer dangerous drugs more quickly. These are needs that cannot be dismissed as cost cuts. Extra nurses on staff results in lives saved (American Nurses Association, 2017), and costs a lot less than multimillion dollar fines and damage to public relations.

Navigators and social workers also have large caseloads, such that they are often unable to spend focused time with individual patients. This is not an effective use of their services. Meeting patients' psychosocial care needs takes time and a thorough, individualized approach. The burden of too much work diminishes care throughout the system.

In addition to care staff, receptionists, schedulers, billing staff, and anyone else who has face-to-face or telephone interactions with patients and their families, affect the patient experience. Every one of these workers must understand that their demeanor impacts patients' outcomes and their ability to heal. Administrators must be willing to take action with problem employees.

7. Money-generating schemes

One tactic in healthcare is to charge facility fees for some newer outpatient facilities (Schulte, 2012). Organizations build freestanding facilities, such as cancer centers, specifically for those services and charge a "facility fee" each time a patient visits for any service. These facility fees can be $200 or more. Whether patients are getting chemotherapy or just having their port flushed, they pay the facility fee. Some insurance companies cover facility fees, but some do not; patients then must pay the fee out-of-pocket. This can add up to thousands of dollars over the course of cancer treatment.

8. Culture

A culture of coercion and fear dominates many healthcare organizations. Care staff do not speak up about safety breaches, violence against healthcare workers, incivility among staff, or unreasonable workloads for fear of being labeled "not a team player"—or worse, being targeted for termination (Hackenthal, 2016). When providers cannot advocate for themselves, they cannot advocate for patients either. Respect, reasonable working conditions, safe patient loads, working equipment, and adequate support staff are required to ensure good outcomes for patients.

In summary, we are losing our way. If we could follow the trail of money, we might learn a lot. We need an aerial view with independent, patient- and public-based oversight to end the siphoning of resources into unknown and unseen pockets away from patient care and healing.

Policymakers and Legislators in Cancer Survivorship

As this is a book about stakeholders in cancer care, I do not dissect policy or healthcare coverage, but I do discuss broad changes that must be made in our legislative process and our culture of healthcare.

National policy and legislation guides what administrators do in the business of healthcare. Legislative influence comes from powerful lobbyists and donors, for whom patients' concerns may not be foremost in their minds.

Legislative bills are voted on by elected officials, many of whom are far removed from the people they impact. Politicians may not know the first thing about healthcare or even their own health. In the U.S., healthcare coverage for legislators far exceeds most ordinary Americans' coverage. They cannot fully empathize with their constituents when they do not experience the same concerns. This impairs their ability to represent the people.

A person's quality of care and coverage can be a matter of life or death in a country that does not provide equal coverage or access to care. Those who receive basic treatment for cancer but do not have access to services to return to full function suffer more from their cancer.

Recent policy and public health initiatives around cancer, along with the uncertainty in health-care legislation, have made it clear that people want health coverage. They do not want to be bankrupted by a system and services that are unevenly and unfairly distributed. Political divisions in the country are making solutions more difficult and contentious, costing lives and quality of life along the way.

Most people, legislators included, do not understand that cancer is not something that happens to somebody else. Its likelihood is high enough that each individual might as well count on it and have a plan for it.

Other Stakeholders in Healthcare

There are many entities involved in cancer care, from government agencies involved in re-search and policy, like the National Institutes of Health; national nonprofit organizations, such as the National Coalition for Cancer Survivorship and the American Cancer Society; public health organizations at the state and local levels; and community-based nonprofits that provide financial and other services after a cancer diagnosis. Fundraising organizations sponsor events for cancer-related causes, and community providers offer complementary care and therapeutic modalities for healing.

These organizations benefit the person with cancer indirectly, by funding research, or directly, by providing financial resources to offset costs and fill the gaps in support, care, and healing. Healthcare organizations should inform patients about their services and be willing to work with community and complementary providers in service of the patient. The future of healthcare reform in the U.S. will guide these organizations, but they will maintain their importance even if single-payer healthcare is adopted. As the healthcare system works with these organizations, the support needs will be met for many more people, and they will experience better quality of life.

Solutions

1. Approach

After the death of his son, Beau, former Vice President Joe Biden was motivated to propose the Biden Cancer Initiative, but something more than a moonshot is needed for big changes to healthcare. Lives are being saved like never before, but what kind of lives are cancer survivors leading after diagnosis and treatment? And for those who are living longer with advanced cancer, what is being done to make their situations more livable?

There must be more research into quality of life, what keeps people healthy, how to change behavior, and how to improve the odds of survival. There must be focus on early detection but also on actions that lower the likelihood of getting sick in the first place. People can learn to take better care of themselves so their bodies will be in better condition for treatment. The money spent on treatment must deliver better health outcomes. People must have access to essential services such as mental health care, which is connected to many physical health issues. Let's put resources at the base, not the tip, of the pyramid.

People must take responsibility for their health, understand the healthcare system, and learn how to self-advocate within it. Healthcare education should be broadened. People must learn to be responsible stewards of healthcare resources and to support greater allocation of resources for mental health services, addiction treatment, and chronic care.

Cancer Harbors (page A16) and the Prevent-Prepare-Prehab curriculum (page A46) address these needs.

2. Averse to risk, averse to progress

We should encourage creativity and innovation in cancer survivorship care with reasonable incentives, recognition, and awards. Innovation must be for the sake of human benefit, however, not for the sake of profit.

3. Community, connection, and communication

Healthcare facilities must end their competition for patients when it leads to wasteful duplication of services. Communities should not permit multiple medical facilities to be built where there is no need. Instead, healthcare organizations should communicate, use resources wisely, and work together to provide for patients' needs.

The investment in duplicate services in one community could be better used to cultivate human resources. Staffing sufficiently, which frees up time for employees providing care, will encourage interdisciplinary collaboration among physicians, nurses, and other professional clinical staff. This should be incorporated into organizational culture.

Moreover, let's arrange social and business networking events for community service providers to establish relationships, awareness, and trust with physicians. All healthcare providers should be allowed time to attend these events to expand their potential referrals. Providers who are knowledgeable about the community are better advocates for patients.

In an industry as fast-paced and automated as healthcare, where everyone is trying to do more with fewer human resources, it is important to remember that balancing on this precarious tightrope takes effort, thought, and judgment, qualities only humans possess. Clinicians are not machines, and patients are not widgets on an assembly line.

4. Leadership

We must show integrity and professionalism when assembling healthcare personnel. Staff at all levels of the organization should hone their people skills. Managers must be held accountable for creating hospitable and supportive working environments, and incivility between employees should not be permitted. An uncomfortable workplace ultimately impacts the patient experience, whether in the exam room or reception.

5. Mental health is inseparable from physical health

Poor mental health is conjoined with nearly all the chronic health conditions and preventable illnesses we see in healthcare facilities. Depression and anxiety are common among cancer patients and their caregivers. To control costs of healthcare, mental health services must be widely accessible. Resolving social problems such as wealth disparity, poverty, lack of education, lack of access to resources and facilities, and unsafe communities will reduce healthcare costs. The president of the American Association for Cancer Research for the 2017-18 term, Michael Caligiuri, MD, lists reducing health disparities as his main goal (Rosenthal, 2017).

6. Qualities of good leadership

Those who lead and make decisions must respect the qualities of creativity, authenticity, resourcefulness, and empathy. Until leaders in healthcare take a more resourceful and creative perspective, there will be no reduction in waste, duplication, and inefficiency. Until healthcare executives exhibit empathy for all—patients and care staff—and are willing to acknowledge their authentic selves, we will not resolve the disparities and shortcomings of the cancer experience.

7. Tools

We already have free tools to help cancer patients: hands, feet, eyes, and ears. Nurses use them all the time, but such simple tools can be a hard sell to leadership. Administrators should use them by shadowing nurses and doctors, listening, following, and lending a hand. They should observe how their mandates impact staff and patients. Until they have seen firsthand what cancer care entails, they have no business being in a leadership position in cancer care. Effective leading requires experience in following.

8. Trust

In cancer care and all healthcare, administrators should not keep secrets from hospital staff. They must be transparent with employees, and invite them to planning sessions to build trust and buy-in. Employees who are included feel more valued. Every healthcare organization should implement a "Take Your Boss to Work Day," wherein the manager listens as employees point out snags in their processes. Creating a bridge between the administrative offices and care staff will enhance the patient experience.

9. Voting

Those in positions of leadership must respect the citizens' power to vote. Voting citizens must elect officials who represent their interests. The problems of wealth disparity and poverty must be solved before we can control costs or resolve gaps in care. Healthcare coverage must be available and accessible to all. We need leaders—whether healthcare executives or elected officials—who are held accountable for their actions. When it comes to healthcare, we are all members of the same party: the human party.

I have written this chapter to present issues that interfere with healthcare professionals' ability to provide the best and safest patient care possible. It is my hope that, as a country, we will realize that our winner-take-all approach to healthcare resources is not serving us well.

In my position, outside any major healthcare organization, I am at liberty to speak my mind without fear of losing my job. By pointing out the shortcomings and providing solutions, I hope to provoke self-reflection among those in the upper echelon, as well as the employees and patients who work for and are served by the current system.

Let's be human-centered, realistic, own our imperfections, and get to work on making a system that benefits everyone.

Calls to Action for Healthcare Administrators

» Healthcare leaders should regard their roles as a service to others. A service mentality among administration would increase transparency, responsibility, and accountability. Good leaders help those they lead rise up.

» Healthcare administrators should stop attempting to control what their employees say through scripting. Patients see right through the scripted language. If administrators do not feel they can trust their employees to say the right thing, they must examine the causes of this lack of trust.

» Administrators and decision-makers should spend time observing how their decisions affect patients and staff. They must step out of their corporate suites and interact with the people behind the numbers. They should be accountable to their employees, even walking in their shoes for a day.

References

Adamopoulos, H. (2014, September 8). Why U.S. hospital administrative costs are among the highest in the world: 7 things to know. *Beckers Hospital Review*. Retrieved April 14, 2017, from https://www.beckershospitalreview.com/finance/why-u-s-hospital-administrative-costs-are-among-the-highest-in-the-world-7-things-to-know.html

American College of Healthcare Executives. (n.d.). *Commitment to ethics*. Retrieved April 14, 2017, from https://www.ache.org/abt_ache/commitment_to_ethics.cfm

American Nurses Association. (2017). *Safe staffing literature review*. Retrieved April 14, 2017, from http://www.nursingworld.org/2014-NurseStaffing-UpdatedLiteratureReview

American Society for Clinical Oncology. (2017). *ASCO principles for patient-centered healthcare reform*. Retrieved April 14, 2017, from https://www.asco.org/advocacy-policy/asco-in-action/asco-releases-principles-patient-centered-healthcare-reform

Begley, S. & Respaut, R. (2013, March 6). Special report: Behind a cancer-treatment firm's rosy survival claims. *Reuters*. Retrieved April 17, 2017, from http://www.reuters.com/article/us-usa-cancer-ctca-idUSBRE9250L820130306

Cameron, W. B. (1967). Informal sociology: A casual introduction to sociological thinking (5th ed.) New York: Random House.

Center for Medicare and Medicaid Services. (2016). *Oncology care model*. Retrieved April 14, 2017, from https://innovation.cms.gov/initiatives/oncology-care/

Hackenthal, V. (2016, April 27). Workplace violence rampant in healthcare. *Medscape Nurses*. Retrieved April 14, 2017, from http://www.medscape.com/viewarticle/862562

Mirza, A. (2017, March 9). Hospitals waste billions of dollars in medical supplies. *U.S. News & World Report*. Retrieved April 19, 2017, from https://www.usnews.com/news/healthcare-of-to-morrow/articles/2017-03-09/hospitals-are-wasting-billions-of-dollars-worth-of-medical-equipment

Rau, J. (2013, March 18). Hospital ratings are in the eye of the beholder. *Kaiser Health News*. Retrieved April 19, 2017, from https://khn.org/news/expanding-number-of-groups-offer-hospital-ratings/

Rosenthal, E. T. (2017, April 9). AACR aims for cancer health equality. *MedPage Today*. Retrieved April 14, 2017, from https://www.medpagetoday.com/MeetingCoverage/AACR/64452?xid=nl_mpt_DHE_2017-04-10&eun=g309257d0r&pos=1

Schulte, F. (2014, May 19). Hospital 'facility fees' boosting medical bills, and not just for hospital care. *Center for Public Integrity*. Retrieved April 19, 2017, from https://www.publicintegrity.org/2012/12/20/11978/hospital-facility-fees-boosting-medical-bills-and-not-just-hospital-care

Chapter Six: Calming the Sea

Meeting patient and caregiver needs

"Finding the cure and healing is what we as people should aspire to. Sadly, looking back, I find the fight is with our healthcare system: doctors, their office staff, the facilities, insurance…"

– Apryl Allen, *A Tango with Cancer: My Perilous Dance with Healthcare and Healing*[1]

There is much to be gained from being informed about cancer before a diagnosis. Anything we do to prepare ourselves might have positive results, whether for ourselves or for a loved one.

Dealing with disease is a process, as is recovery. You are not informed of that at the outset of a cancer diagnosis, and certainly not before you ever get sick. There is a social stigma around illness, so we rarely discuss it. But stigmatization makes it more difficult for people to cope when they are faced with illness themselves.

The war metaphors and battle clichés used in fundraisers, the media, obituaries, and everyday conversations are a convenient emotional framework for cancer. They are shortcuts to help us avoid thinking deeply about the subject. We need to give up the shortcuts and tear-jerker sound-bites and have a serious conversation about illness instead.

Cancer will affect 38 percent of us personally in our lifetimes (National Cancer Institute, 2017), and nearly everyone not affected directly will be impacted as caregivers or supporters. Knowing how to cope with cancer as a patient or a caregiver is a universally needed skill.

There is no better source of information than someone who has experienced cancer firsthand. Cancer survivors should be visible and vocal, but they are still often hidden because of our desire to deny the disease's prevalence. Billboards for cancer centers feature healthy-looking

---

1   Allen, 2016, p. 203

bald people, but this is an unnatural and unrealistic representation of people with cancer. They may feel and look unwell. We must accept them as they are and ask to hear from them.

We need to stop hiding cancer; to hide something so prevalent is to live in denial. Statistically, we all should expect to have cancer or another serious illness at some point in our lives. This is pragmatism, not pessimism.

We must stop thinking that health and cancer are mutually exclusive; they can exist together. Cancer frequently happens to people who take good care of themselves. And many patients, as you will read later in this chapter, continue to lead healthy lives while being treated for cancer.

We must pull ourselves out of denial and prepare ourselves to live—and live well—during and after cancer. Two-thirds of cancer survivors now live beyond five years after diagnosis (National Cancer Institute, 2017), which was unimaginable a short while ago. There are greater numbers of people living longer with Stage IV, or metastatic cancer, than ever before. We must include them in our considerations of living with optimal quality.

Recovery from cancer is a process, often lifelong, with no distinct end. Still, most people want to feel closure and that their state of illness is ending. Some are able to view the cancer experience as unfinished and accept their lack of control without experiencing ongoing anxiety. It can take years to achieve this level of peace. The point is to find a way to function and enjoy a quality life, even if even if you can never be free of the burden of cancer.

In this chapter, I discuss the needs of cancer patients with the intent to spare them many of the difficulties people often experience. I explain the role of survivorship care plans, along with their drawbacks, and I explain the Cancer Harbors approach to post-treatment care and referrals. Then I discuss the role patients can play in changing our approach to cancer care.

Before I do so, I provide an overview of the Cancer Harbors program, which is referenced and linked to throughout the text.

The Cancer Harbors Program for Survivors

The Cancer Harbors program provides cancer patients with instructions on navigating beyond treatment in ways that prioritize health and quality of life. The appendix of this book contains a portion of the Cancer Harbors modules (page A16). Links to the rest of the Cancer Harbors modules are available at https://cancerharbors.com/table-of-contents-cancer-harbors/.

The Cancer Harbors program addresses six main areas of gaps in knowledge, skills, and resources among people diagnosed with cancer:

» Navigating the healthcare system while addressing holistic recovery needs and aftereffects of cancer treatment

» Physical activity, nutrition, weight control, and health behaviors to reduce risk of recurrence

» Self-care and restoration, healing environments, therapeutic creativity, spirituality, intimacy, and sexuality

» Mental and emotional health, communication and support, setting limits and boundaries, facing fears, and clarifying values

» Self-advocacy, health, media and consumer literacy, and learning

» Cognitive, occupational, personal, and social growth, setting realistic goals, moving forward, and identification of resources for future needs

The skills taught in Cancer Harbors are useful even if you do not have cancer, and they provide excellent preparation for a future encounter with the healthcare system. All readers of this book, including healthcare professionals, can benefit from the Cancer Harbors program.

Gaps in the Process

This section examines how people in healthcare—namely, patients and providers—approach the cancer process. I will relate patients' stories to identify problems and solutions, and I will identify Cancer Harbors lessons to close these gaps in care.

Gaps in cancer care can occur along the entire timeline of a patient's experience. It's best to break the process down chronologically: before treatment, during treatment, and after treatment. After I review the process, I will identify solutions for improvement.

Before Treatment

Before treatment, a patient receives a diagnosis, the result of a series of tests and procedures to identify the type of cancer. This diagnosis is often met with varying degrees of shock, paralysis, and fear.

Asking the right questions

It is difficult to make sense of the diagnosis, or even to know what questions to ask. "Am I going to die?" is often the first question. While legitimate, the question is driven by fear, loss of control, and the unknown. More practical questions would be:

» What do I need to do to prepare for this?

» What do I do first?

» What can wait?

» What do I need right now?

» Who can I talk to?

» Who can I trust with this information?

» Who can I rely on?

At this time (or, ideally, before a diagnosis) patients should establish their values and set up contingency plans, which includes naming a designated advocate and caregiver they trust. This can allow patients to maintain a sense of control until they are ready to step back into the driver's seat. Choosing an advocate is a necessary step, though it can be a difficult conversation to initiate. (See the Prevent-Prepare-Prehab section on page A46 for additional information on values, advocates, and caregivers.)

The need for answers is foremost in the mind of the person just diagnosed with cancer. Patients need to know why, how, what, when, where, what-if, and what-if-I-don't in response to countless questions. A list of questions patients may wish to ask their doctors begins on the next page.

Questions to ask your doctor if you are diagnosed with cancer

» Why are you suggesting this treatment option?

» What generally happens as this disease progresses?

» What are the goals for my care? Can the cancer be cured, or just controlled?

» What are the risks and benefits of the treatments I am being offered?

» What are the advantages and disadvantages of each option, in the short term and long term?

» How much does each one cost?

» How will each affect both my quality of life and length of life?

» How long am I likely to live if I do, or if I don't, get treated?

» How does this treatment work on the cancer in my body?

» Are there less toxic options available?

» What will happen to me if I don't take this treatment?

» How many patients have you given this treatment regimen to? What happened to their cancer? How are they doing now?

» What are the side effects during treatment?

» What help will I have available to me to control the side effects or symptoms that come from the treatment?

» What are the lasting effects after treatment, and how long will I be affected?

» What are some possible late effects (10, 20, 30 years from now)?

» Will I need additional medications or treatments after this treatment is done?

» If this treatment doesn't work, what would you recommend?

» Do people ever decide to stop getting this treatment? What happens to them? In what situations would you recommend that this treatment be stopped?

» What can I do to succeed in getting through treatment?

» What resources can you refer me to for support? (e.g., physical/occupational/ speech therapy, exercise programs, nutritional counseling, mental health care)

» What can I do to reduce the chances the cancer will return? Or, what can I do in the face of advanced disease and an uncertain or limited prognosis?

Questions to ask your doctor if you are diagnosed with cancer *(continued)*

» What can I do to recover my pre-diagnosis way of life? (This requires that you let your doctor know who you are, what is important to you, and your personal values.)

» How can I maximize my quality of life regardless of changes? Or, if the cancer is very advanced and the treatments are not curative, how can I maximize my quantity and quality of life in the time I have left?

» Will you and your team be there for me after treatment? What is your approach to meeting my needs?

» How hard will it be for me to recover from this? What kind of work will I need to do after treatment to get back to where I was before I got sick?

» If you don't know how to answer some of my questions, will you refer me to someone who can help me?

More questions can be found in the Cancer Harbors modules on self-advocacy at https://cancerharbors.com/table-of-contents-cancer-harbors/.

Information can be anxiety-provoking, but anxiety worsens with too little or too much information. Patients want to feel some control over their situation, or at least have some certainty for what is about to happen. The more anxiety they have, the less they are able to absorb. At initial diagnosis, many patients try to rely on their doctors to make decisions and tell them what to do.

Patients must make decisions based on information they have been given and not feel guilty about their choices. But when patients are in shock, experiencing acute anxiety, or grieving the loss of their health, they are not able to process information like they normally would.

That is why patients need advocates—to ask the level-headed questions and remember or record the answers. Patients will reach a point where they can absorb information and formulate questions, but that time may not come until they are well into treatment.

<u>Know your values</u>

Knowing one's values is critical when making such important decisions. The Values Exercise (page A8) can help patients decide which values are most important to them. This will guide them in choosing treatments based on how the outcome aligns with their values. They must be clear about what outcomes they expect from their care; then they can discuss with their providers whether their expectations are realistic.

Trust in doctors

Authenticity, honesty, and full disclosure by doctors is important to gaining patients' trust. Doctors must be honest about the consequences of their life-saving treatments; they must not minimize the adverse effects of treatment and overstate the benefits (Hoffmann & Delmar, 2017). Patients may even want to ask their doctor if they have a tendency to do that.

Patients want hope, but false hope based on incomplete information can cause them to feel betrayed by their doctors. When patients do not trust their doctors, they are vulnerable to armchair oncologists (people who do not have a medical degree but freely give advice on cancer treatment) and snake oil salesmen (people who tout the miracle cures and too-good-to-be true healing properties of a product they are selling).

Patients should get a second opinion if they do not feel good about their doctors, the recommended treatments, or if they have a rare type of cancer. When entrusting a doctor with their future, they should trust their gut.

Despite the importance and benefits for everyday life, it is rare for people to prepare themselves for cancer before a diagnosis. Why is this? Let's look at four of these reasons.

1. Unwillingness to address our mortality

   A cancer diagnosis eliminates this luxury. Most people do not discuss death and do not arrange advance directives; they don't see death as a part of life. Being unprepared for death has social and financial implications for everyone, however, especially loved ones. Addressing your own death in advance is a gift to your loved ones, as they will not have to bear the burden of making difficult decisions while grieving.

   Everyone should be able to face their own mortality; after all, death runs in every family, without exception! We have extended life expectancy through advances in public health, but we are not each guaranteed a long, healthy life.

Many of us feel entitled to 80 or more years of life and feel cheated if we get less. Some people see death as a failure, and the medical community has contributed to this viewpoint for a long time.

2. Inadequate knowledge, motivation, and skills to prevent chronic disease

There is little education about cancer except the importance of screening. Primary care providers often lack time to educate patients on cancer prevention, but they do make sure patients are screened. Health education in schools, if it exists at all, does not address cancer.

3. Inadequate knowledge of one's own body and how it should be functioning

The process of acquiring physical fitness teaches people how to listen to their body. They know what is normal for them. People who know their bodies also know when something is wrong. They may (though not always) be more likely to seek treatment sooner, which usually results in better outcomes.

Further, if they know how they normally function and cancer treatment sets them back, they are more likely to request therapy to restore their previous level of functioning. They are less likely to accept a compromised state or will be more motivated to improve it.

4. Lack of adequate health literacy, science literacy, media literacy, and consumer literacy skills

Low health literacy does not mean uneducated; we cannot be experts on everything. But when patients do not understand the healthcare system or science and do not trust medicine, they are vulnerable and at a disadvantage. These concepts can be explained simply by skilled educators. For example, a nurse advocate has written an excellent blog post (Llewellyn, 2015) on how the process works behind the scenes between patients, doctors, and insurance.

During Treatment

Gaps in care occur throughout treatment as well. They are often related to securing support and resources.

<u>Coping with anxiety</u>

Patients may have heard horror stories about the side effects of chemotherapy or other treatments and have terrible anxiety going into their first treatment session. A good nurse can educate patients and will explain what they will experience, how it will feel, and how they are likely to respond during and after the treatment session. Most of the time, it is not as bad as the patient imagined.

Patients should be informed, however, that the effects of chemotherapy add up over time. They will feel progressively more tired and experience more side effects during the weeks or months of treatment. This is the clichéd "battle" phase, but it is quite the passive battlefield—sitting in a chair and letting the chemo drip into a port, or lying on a table painlessly being irradiated—until several weeks go by, and the effects start to accumulate.

Patients can use distraction to lower anxiety. After the first few treatments, they will know what to expect and what they like during a treatment, whether it is having a companion, sleeping, watching TV, reading, or another activity that passes the time.

A book or resource about what to expect in chemotherapy, such as *Getting Past the Fear* by Nancy Stordahl (2014), can also be very helpful.

Supportive care

During chemotherapy treatment, the side effects can be minimized with careful use of medications to control nausea or other symptoms. This goal of symptom management and optimizing quality of life during treatment is called supportive care. Supportive care, also known as palliative care, is slowly becoming more accepted for patients undergoing curative treatment. (For further discussion on palliative care, refer to page 31.)

Home health care

During treatment, patients with temporary functional impairments can make use of home health care services until their independence is restored. Medicare covers home health services, and some private insurers also cover it. Doctors often do not refer eligible patients for home care, but it is much less expensive than the facility fees for hospitals and outpatient cancer centers.

Insurance

During treatment, many patients need help working with insurance companies. The fight is made even more difficult because the patient is tired, unwell, and does not have the cognitive focus to take on this frustrating task. Usually, patients begin receiving bills for their care while they are still undergoing treatment.

A person who is knowledgeable about insurance companies and billing is an excellent resource. Bills can be negotiated, perhaps saving a patient thousands of dollars. Likewise, pharmaceutical companies offer programs for reduced-cost drugs, but many people are unaware of these programs.

Patient advocates may be able to help navigate these tasks. The Patient Advocate Foundation (http://patientadvocate.org/) is a good place to start. Financial coaches and counselors can be found in some localities. Use caution with anyone you hire; make sure they are reputable.

Patient safety

The body is in a state of disequilibrium when going through cancer treatment, and adverse effects are highly likely to occur. When safety slips through the cracks, it is usually because of a lack of communication or understanding. Both patients and caregivers must be educated on how to respond when they have concerning symptoms. They should be informed about when to call the oncologist, to use urgent care, or to go to the emergency department.

Communication with other medical personnel

Patients and caregivers cannot assume that medical personnel outside their oncologist's office will be familiar with their treatment regimen or even know they are being treated for cancer. When patients go to the emergency department (ED), for example, they or their caregiver must communicate the cancer diagnosis and treatment to the treating physician. Some forward-thinking facilities are providing cancer patients with an alert card to present upon admission to the ED, so staff will initiate the necessary precautions.

After Treatment and the Gaps in Survivorship Care Plans

Despite widespread recommendations for the use of survivorship care plans, gaps in care occur after treatment, too, even as a result of the plans.

What are survivorship care plans?

The survivorship care plan (SCP) is the current approach to meet the ongoing needs of cancer patients after treatment. The SCP provides a treatment summary, indicators of recurrence, a schedule of follow-up screenings, potential long-term effects of treatment, and healthy lifestyle guidelines.

Survivorship care plans were proposed in 2005 in the report *Lost in Transition: From Cancer Patient to Cancer Survivor*, which brought to light the numerous and long-lasting aftereffects of cancer treatment for which patients were not receiving support (Institute of Medicine, 2005). These plans were originally intended to help people recover and manage their health after cancer treatment, and as a guideline for follow-up care.

After cancer treatment, the patient's primary care provider usually resumes caring for the patient, except in matters directly related to the cancer. Communication between primary care providers and oncologists is not consistent, however, and not every patient receives an SCP. The American College of Surgeons Commission on Cancer (2016) has recommended 50% of all patients receive SCPs by the end of 2017, with 100% compliance recommended by 2019.[2]

One answer to this recommendation is the Oncology Care Model (OCM) of 2016 (Centers for Medicare and Medicaid Services, 2016). It established requirements that providers of oncology services must meet to be reimbursed by Medicare or commercial insurers. The OCM sets a standard for oncology practices to "provide higher quality, more coordinated oncology care," which includes requiring a care plan that considers quality of life and psychosocial issues. This ensures that patients receive SCPs, but it does not fix the current shortcomings of SCPs, which will be addressed in a later section.

Several entities have developed templates for SCPs. The American Society of Clinical Oncology (ASCO, 2014) and the Livestrong Foundation (http://livestrongcareplan.org) provide two commonly used plans. The plans take differing perspectives, with ASCO's template focusing on the follow-up needs of medical professionals, and Livestrong's plan presenting questions from the patient's point of view.

ASCO's template is basic and objective, developed by medical professionals for their use. It summarizes the patient's diagnosis and treatment and providers who were involved. It contains a recommended schedule for follow-up visits, framing the patient's survivorship care as an ongoing series of follow-up screenings, scans, labs, and visits for early detection of recurrence. It details the likely and unlikely long-term effects the patient might experience after treatment. It also contains general information for common psychosocial issues that may concern the patient and provides basic guidelines for a healthy lifestyle.

---

2 As of December 11, 2017, the Commission on Cancer has made downward adjustments to these mandates, requiring only 50% compliance for eligible patients in 2018. There may be future adjustments after the printing of this book.

The Livestrong Foundation's plan is less clinical in its approach, presented from the point of view of the patient. It covers the same topics around recovery and post-treatment psychosocial concerns. Though the Livestrong plan may be more appealing to the patient, it has shortcomings similar to other SCPs. According to Daudt et al. (2014), it may not include a consistent point of contact for ongoing coordination of care, nor provide comprehensive psychosocial support resources.

Shortcomings of survivorship care plans

There are several drawbacks and criticisms of SCPs, which lead to gaps in care. First, SCPs are convenient for physicians because they provide a pre-planned approach, but this may cause healthcare professionals to take a narrow view of follow-up care. The patient's personal characteristics, lifestyle, and other factors mean recovery and everyday life is more complex than can be captured in a linear plan.

SCPs specify follow-up medical visits and other tests for prevention or detection of recurrence, considering only the patient's medical needs. They do not provide a suggested care process for complementary or outside providers. They medicalize cancer patients' post-treatment experiences, rather than encouraging them to normalize their lives.

While the SCP gives patients general guidelines on practicing healthy behaviors such as exercising, eating nutritious foods, wearing sunscreen, and sticking to their follow-up plan and preventive screenings, it gives no specific guidance on developing these self-care skills. Patients who never engaged in these positive behaviors before diagnosis may be at a loss to start now.

Further, certain services, when coded as rehabilitation, are covered by insurance. Thus, medical centers gain revenue from patients who are referred to in-house clinical facilities for services that may be billed as rehab, such as exercise and nutrition. Many patients, however, do not need rehab and instead should be encouraged to seek support from community providers.

There is also little data on the effectiveness of SCPs in improving long-term outcomes, reducing recurrence, lowering healthcare costs, or improving quality of life (Brennan, Gormally, Butow, Boyle, & Spillane, 2014; Daudt et al., 2014). These gaps in evidence might diminish the longer SCPs are in use. Daudt et al. (2014) provide a review of SCP use in various countries and point out the lack of consistency in following Institute of Medicine guidelines.

Another drawback to traditional SCPs is the trauma they can induce in patients. During the counseling session to present the SCP, patients are reminded of the risks of recurrence. They are fearful of leaving their oncologists' careful watch, and they are learning about (or being reminded of) all the potential adverse effects of treatment.

Moreover, the Commission on Cancer's directives for providing SCPs also miss an important group of patients. They do not include those with metastatic disease for whom cure is not possible (American College of Surgeons Commission on Cancer, 2016), but late-stage cancer patients are alive, desiring quality of life, and should not be forgotten. Even if their physicians cannot provide life-saving treatment for their cancer, these patients have real, everyday needs for supportive care.

Finally, and most problematic, is the unpredictability of survivorship services needed following treatment. As each patient and situation differ, so do the issues that surface in the months and years following treatment for cancer. While many survivors experience most aftereffects (such as fatigue, acute anxiety, and lingering treatment effects) within a short period of time after treatment, others may not experience serious needs related to their cancer experience for many years after treatment has ended.

At the outset of survivorship, doctors cannot predict their patients' needs for the post-treatment period. Likewise, survivors have no idea what the future holds. In essence, they don't know what they don't know.

Thus, a one-size-fits-all approach is not suited to survivorship care planning. The approach to survivorship care must be flexible to manage issues and needs for support over time.

The Cancer Harbors Plan

Cancer Harbors was developed out of the need for a more thoughtful approach to survivorship after treatment. It complements the doctor's guidelines for follow-up care after treatment, whether that is provided in an SCP or some other form.

Cancer Harbors is a practical program, focusing on the real-life, everyday functional needs of cancer survivors that often go unaddressed during follow-up doctor appointments. It enables participants to balance their expectations and desire to quickly return to full function and health, with understanding of the comprehensive nature of healing after cancer treatment.

Cancer Harbors takes into account that our struggles around cancer are not simple—they have complex physical, emotional, social, and spiritual sources—and helps build self-care skills to resolve them.

As the survivor transitions from the constant watch of their clinical team during the acute phase of treatment, it encourages the patient to take more control over their health choices and to find resources to further their recovery.

Participants have expressed the benefits of the Cancer Harbors program to their lives in these words:

> "I was unprepared for what recovery from cancer would entail and how long it would take. Cancer Harbors allowed me to stop focusing on how long it will take, and instead, on growing from where I am now, with what I have at this moment. This allowed me to reduce my anxiety and enjoy life rather than focusing on what I couldn't do. Eventually, I was able to do everything I'd done before cancer, and more."

> "I have experienced a personal transformation and grown emotionally and spiritually, as well as gaining knowledge I wish I'd had before I had cancer."

> "While the physicians saved my life, Cancer Harbors made life more enjoyable."

> "I did not have confidence in my body after my diagnosis—it betrayed me. I needed to regain my health and my self-confidence."

> "The uncertainty about the future can be overwhelming, but Cancer Harbors helps me to not focus on the uncertainty, and instead, build my strength and skills, in all different areas of my life, to make me more resilient to anything that might come my way in the future. The resources and creativity that are contained in this program are unlike anything else."

> "After feeling like a number in the medical world, it is a refreshing, personal, and genuine twist on meeting my recovery needs."

> "It has taught me not to be defined by my illness."

Post-treatment Concerns

Many patients who experience long-lasting aftereffects of treatment are hesitant to report problems to their doctor; they do not want to be labeled a chronic complainer or hypochondriac. But when their bodies have betrayed them with cancer, small issues can create great anxiety about recurrence until they adjust to their post-treatment body.

The concerns most reported by cancer survivors during and after treatment are fatigue, cognitive impairment, and loss of social or medical support (Naughton & Weaver, 2014). Late effects and the need for referrals to other medical or non-medical providers are also post-treatment concerns for patients.

1. Fatigue

There are many causes of fatigue: physical, psychological, environmental, and others. Initially, when recovering from surgeries, chemotherapy, or radiation, the body needs to heal and uses much energy for this cause. It takes months, for example, for bone marrow to recover and replace the red blood cells that carry oxygen to the tissues, healing the condition called anemia.

Depression and anxiety also contribute to fatigue, as well as cognitive impairment. Readjusting to work or family obligations, managing bills and financial stress, and keeping up with social demands can be exhausting. Other reasons, such as impaired thyroid function or nutritional deficiencies, may also contribute to fatigue after treatment.

There is a growing body of evidence that exercise is the most effective way to relieve fatigue (Mustian et al, 2017). Physical activity improves recovering patients' ability to enjoy life and be healthy, and it reduces their chances of a cancer recurrence. Barriers to participating in exercise are prevalent, however, and they can be difficult to overcome. These barriers include low self-confidence, intimidation, lack of knowledge, lack of social support, lack of a safe environment, lack of time or child care, or inability to afford gyms, equipment, or clothing.

Patients should request a referral to a physical or occupational therapist if impairments in function are inhibiting their quality of life post-treatment. Physical or occupational therapy may help patients improve their physical abilities to the point where they can reap the health benefits from physical activity. Insight and guidance from a skilled provider make this transition easier. When patients have completed rehab, then can benefit greatly from a supportive community program such as FIERCE.

(The FIERCE program, described in the appendix, was developed to address many of these barriers. It is a supportive, noncompetitive learning environment that emphasizes movement and activity. A Cancer Harbors module called "Coping with Fatigue" can be found at https://cancerharbors.com/table-of-contents-cancer-harbors/.)

2. Cognitive impairment

For a long time, doctors dismissed complaints of "chemo brain"—difficulty with concentration, memory, attention, or other aspects of cognitive function—because there were no data to support it as a condition. Now we know cognitive difficulties persist after treatment (National Cancer Institute, 2017).

Neurocognitive research has shown that chemicals called cytokines are released by the immune system when there is inflammation in the body caused by disease, treatment, or the process of healing (Kesler, 2013). Some cytokines fight the inflammation, but others may contribute to the feeling of brain fog (Bower et al, 2013).

Evidence is needed to help solve these unintended effects of treatment, but this can still be a blind spot for doctors. Patients should not allow their concerns to be dismissed. Some people may have a genetic pre-disposition to produce more of these chemicals, which contributes to the worsening of cognitive performance (Bower et al., 2013).

(For more information on cognitive impairment, see the Cancer Harbors module titled "What To Do About Chemo Brain and Cognitive Dysfunction" at https://cancerharbors.com/table-of-contents-cancer-harbors/.)

3. Loss of support

Many patients report a loss of support immediately following treatment. Friends and family, who had brought meals, made visits, or run errands, suddenly disappear when the appointments are over. They may mistakenly expect the patient to pick up where he or she left off with everyday work, social, and family activities, not understanding that recovery takes time.

Simultaneously, patients have lost the constant watch of their cancer treatment team. This can contribute to anxiety and a sense of isolation, and it impacts patients' mental health. Janelsins et al. (2016) suggest that by treating anxiety and depression before cancer treatment, people may experience less cognitive impairment, with reduced impact on quality of life.

Destigmatizing mental health needs is key. No one should be expected to handle cancer without experiencing depression or anxiety. Further, it can be treated and relieved, making cancer and all its traumas seem less overwhelming.

(Refer to the module, "Trauma, PTSD, and Coping," at https://cancerharbors.com/table-of-contents-cancer-harbors/ for more on loss of support and mental health impacts.)

4. Late effects

Some patients experience "late effects," which occur many years after cancer treatment (Naughton & Weaver, 2014). Possible late effects include the development of new cancers, especially of the bone marrow, as well as permanent damage to organs or tissue, disability, or loss of function. They pose a greater problem for cancer survivors who will live 20 or more years beyond treatment. Patients need support while learning to live a quality life with late effects.

5. Requesting referrals

Doctors do not see the everyday functional impairments, struggles, anxiety, fatigue, and social, sexual, and cognitive difficulties, or how they affect relationships and social and occupational functioning. Do not think your doctor is too busy. Minimizing your complaints is a sure way to avoid getting the care you need.

Doctors may not have all the answers, and service providers in the community can fill in gaps in recovery. Physicians should make referrals and encourage patients to continually seek help in recovering, but patients may also need to request referrals.

Patients must acknowledge for themselves that recovery is a long process, that they need help coping, and that they deserve that help. Patients are happier when they have a chance to find relief. Survivors do not come out the other side of cancer treatment unchanged.

The Patient Experience

I frequently speak to cancer support groups in my community. I ask, "What do you wish you had known before this happened?" Usually they respond, "I wish I had known what to ask when the doctor said, 'Do you have any questions for me?'"

Cancer survivors also did not realize they would need to be their own advocates. They needed help in that role, as they were completely unprepared for it. Too many times, survivors have bemoaned, "You are just a number in the medical world."

Several patients mentioned the massive folder of information given to them, a folder they never looked at again. They said, "It would have been nice to know all the adverse effects. They give you lots of material to read but don't explain it and leave it up to you to figure it out."

I designed the materials in this book for both cancer survivors as well as those who have never had cancer but may become advocates. Whether you are reeling from your own cancer diagnosis or you are assisting someone recently diagnosed, you will be better informed to ask questions or make care decisions.

Let's look at some patients' stories and how their experiences could be directed to create change. Names and personal details have been changed to protect their privacy.

Joe's Story

Joe was 59 and a healthy ultra distance runner when he began to experience increasing fatigue over a period of a year. He was diagnosed with myeloma, a blood cancer that affects the kidneys, bones, and other organs.

He had endured a lengthy hospitalization a few years earlier due to a foot infection and sepsis, followed by an extended stay in a rehabilitation facility to regain his strength. He had recovered and returned to running ultramarathons (races longer than a standard 26-mile marathon) not long before his cancer diagnosis.

Joe initially received oral chemotherapy, and his response indicated that he was a good candidate for an autologous stem cell transplant. In this procedure, healthy precursor cells that make mature blood cells were harvested from his own bone marrow and re-infused into his body after a strong dose of chemotherapy, which killed off his remaining stem cells. This procedure is like a reboot of the bone marrow; it gets rid of the cancerous stem cells and prompts the bone marrow to resume normal cell production.

It is a complicated process, and his body had no immunity until his bone marrow replaced his blood cells. He was hospitalized for several weeks after the transplant and then spent a period of isolation in an apartment near the hospital until his immune system was strong enough for him to go home. This is normal procedure in a transplant of this type.

"Going through the process," Joe recounted, "was like going through a car wash—a wave of information washes over you and rolls off like water. There's no way to absorb all that information" (personal communication, April 5, 2017).

His wife was with him as an advocate. She asked questions and kept track of the information. She and Joe are knowledgeable and well-educated. She could filter through a lot of the junk online to find good supplemental information. Joe was lucky to have a supportive boss and job situation, and he took off as much time as he needed and worked from home when able.

"It hit my wife like a ton of bricks. For me, I saw it as just another ultra. I'll do what I can and try to get across the finish line," he said, acknowledging that not everything was under his control (personal communication, April 5, 2017).

Mental toughness and endurance were assets for Joe. Doctors were not particularly forthcoming with information, so he had to ask many questions. He did not always know what to ask, however. Doctors never mentioned mental health care, but they had plenty of information on topics like avoiding infection.

Joe found it annoying that his healthcare providers did not understand him as an athlete. He has low blood pressure and a low resting heart rate from being so physically fit, but they retook his blood pressure constantly and would call the doctor, concerned, even though he told them his low blood pressure readings were normal.

He learned years before during his hospitalization with sepsis that he must be as active and strong as possible going into treatment. He ran the entire time he was taking oral chemotherapy, lowering his intensity of effort when he was anemic, but continuing his workouts. He also "trained" for his stem cell transplant, knowing that the better shape he was in, the less likely he would be to have problems.

He now stays on a maintenance dose of chemotherapy with frequent follow-ups to keep an eye on the cancer's status. There are no guarantees, but he has returned to running ultramarathons.

Sandy's Story

Sandy, a mother of young children, was diagnosed with Stage IV cervical cancer. She sees that good health can co-exist with cancer. "I am not a disease. I have a disease, but I am not a disease. You cannot just manage my disease. I am a whole person" (personal communication, January 20, 2017).

Sandy was diagnosed by an ob-gyn doctor she no longer sees after months of complaining about pelvic pain that was not resolved. Upon being given the news, she was not referred to any sort of counseling or mental health support. She was in crisis and needed help immediately.

When she called me about her diagnosis, I urged her to see a counselor right away, even before she saw her new oncologist.

Sandy had an excellent experience with her oncologist and the facility where she was treated. Upon talking to other cancer survivors, however, she heard about experiences that were different from her own. "I was surprised. I had a great experience, but I didn't realize that's not everyone's experience" (personal communication, January 20, 2017).

She felt that mental health support should be emphasized, along with physical therapy and other services. "They have those departments there for a reason, right? They need to get them used. In my mind, it wasn't optional. Mental health is not optional. It's all part of dealing with this!" (personal communication, January 20, 2017).

About her late-stage diagnosis, she says, "[I] was talked down to by tons of doctors. I feel like I paid attention to my own instincts leading up to my diagnosis and that's the only reason why I'm alive today" (personal communication, January 20, 2017).

Apryl's Story

Apryl is a musician, business executive, and author who was diagnosed with early stage breast cancer. During treatment, she experienced intense stress in interactions with office personnel and when handling paperwork and insurance claims.

In her book, *A Tango with Cancer: My Perilous Dance with Healthcare and Healing*, she reflected, "Is nobody thoughtful?" (Allen, 2016, p. 287).

She cited the patient and family's need to put energy into healing, not into anxiety-provoking situations. Doctors' and staff's voices have an emotional effect on the patient. She suggested that everyone who works in healthcare be educated in what she calls "the human aspects of an illness—anxiety, fear, and pain" (2016, p. 309). Furthermore, she recommended that healthcare workers—professional and their administrative staff—maintain a "stable and stress-free work environment" (2016, p. 309).

She observed that many of the healthcare workers and staff with whom she interacted seemed to be controlling and compulsive. She could see that they were overworked and understaffed, but her interactions were often unpleasant.

She described the repetitive paperwork and intake process for each appointment. "Introduce yourself," she suggested for reception staff. "'My name is ___ and if you need anything while you're waiting, please raise the flag on this door,' or something!" (Allen, personal communication, April 28, 2017).

She also cited the feeling of being taken hostage once inside the office. Patients are often subject to long waits with no communication from the staff. "You're at their mercy, and you're labeled a difficult patient if you speak up" (personal communication, April 28, 2017).

The lack of privacy in the office waiting areas and the presence of TVs contributed to her discomfort. "Can't they have places where you don't have to listen to the blaring TV?"

There is too much waiting, she noted. "Insurance companies are impersonal, you have to wait an inordinate amount of time for authorizations, and there is no smooth process." Patients are also kept in suspense waiting for results. "The moment the results are received, that should become their number one priority—inform the patient. This is also known as communication" (personal communication, April 28, 2017).

With so many new terms, procedures, and appointments, it is easy for patients to lose track of what each is for. It would help to know the plan. She said, "The patient needs a plan from the beginning. What do I need, and in what order do I need to do it? There's no guidebook, map, or rules for the patient." Apryl was not even given the proper instructions to prepare for her PET scan (personal communication, April 28, 2017).

"How are you supposed to know what questions to ask if you've never experienced something like this?" She added, "It's very stressful on the spouse." No mental health or counseling services were recommended for her and her husband (personal communication, April 28, 2017).

She was not told how to find relief from the pain of radiation, nor was lymphedema discussed. Her surgeon did not tell her about physical therapy after surgery. "Some patients might know to ask about exercises, but what if they don't know?" (personal communication, April 28, 2017)

Staff should listen when patients speak up. Apryl was allergic to certain kinds of tape, which she mentioned, but the wrong type of tape was used on her skin, causing a painful reaction.

Apryl also talked about the need for continuity of care and the importance of patients building relationships with their doctors. "Compassion plays a big role in healing," she said (personal communication, April 28, 2017).

If a patient without a medical background can plainly see so many issues, something is clearly wrong. The following patient-driven solutions may improve cancer care.

Patient-Driven Solutions

1. Give feedback to the healthcare system

For Joe, Sandy, and Apryl, a feedback mechanism would have helped them express concerns and issues to their healthcare teams. Presently, the best feedback mechanism we have is the survey patients often receive from their healthcare facility following a visit. Many people discard them, but they can provide valuable feedback for the specific department. Alternatively, patients may write an evaluation letter and send it directly to the administration or relevant department manager.

Patients may wish to ask whether the institution has a procedure to accept and act upon feedback before they receive treatment there (if they have a choice). If they have a complaint, they should ask to be contacted by someone at the facility. Firsthand stories, emotion, and tone of voice provide more convincing feedback about the situation.

These days, healthcare facilities worry about patient satisfaction. Many patients resort to social media to report difficulties with hospitals or insurance companies, as the last thing a company wants is unsatisfactory public relations in public view. Patients are more likely to get a response if they follow through tactfully but uncompromisingly.

2. Be kind to yourself

Patients need not be stoic; they should ask for help when needed. No one expects patients to be medical experts, and they should not try to be.

When people reach out, do not automatically reply, "I'm fine;" be honest if you are comfortable doing so. When others ask how they can help, think about what you need. Allow yourself to receive help as a gift.

Further, understand how patient support and palliation can help. They are an essential part of care, regardless of the stage of the disease. It is okay to seek relief. Our cultural tendency to be individualistic and self-reliant works to our disadvantage when we are sick. Not accepting or reaching out for help impairs healing and recovery.

Maly, Liang, Liu, Griggs, & Ganz (2017) found that a one-hour counseling session helped people with adherence to their survivorship care plan. What if we provided more than one hour? What if were generous with our care?

3. Be heard, be visible

Patients should be encouraged to interact with the community and share their cancer stories. Cancer is not shameful, and it should not be stigmatized. Others may learn if we remove the shroud of secrecy and mystery.

Patients can speak to support groups and healthcare executives, or share experiences at conferences for doctors and nurses. They can push for patients' voices in medical education. They can participate in Twitter chats, Facebook groups, and blogs. They can also talk to their local, state, and national representatives to express concerns. It is helpful to suggest solutions whenever possible.

Patients may visit community health fairs organized by their hospitals and find the CEO or other top executives, who often make an appearance. They can request time to talk with them. CEOs cannot avoid face-to-face anecdotes, and real faces with stories make a greater impact than numbers on a survey.

4. Lose your fear

Challenging authority is a learned skill. Accepting criticism is also a skill. As a patient, whomever you are talking to should be able to handle criticism; a red flag should be raised in your mind if they cannot. Assert yourself calmly, and insist on answers or being sent in a productive direction.

5. Remember CARE: creativity, authenticity, resourcefulness, and empathy

Patients should expect these qualities from their doctors and all those with whom they interact in healthcare. Doctors and staff should be respectful of patients' time, be willing to try different approaches, and be flexible in their thought processes. They should simply listen.

They must relate to their patients as human beings by acknowledging their own humanity and presenting their real selves.

6. Rethink your role as patient

The word "patient" carries a connotation of passivity and submission to the all-knowing, all-powerful doctor in an antiquated, paternalistic system. We are no longer living in those times. Patients can be active, informed participants in decision-making around their health and their futures.

The Cancer Harbors and FIERCE programs in the appendix contain a wealth of material to match the resources patients need to the issues they are facing. They help patients build the skills they need to cope more effectively.

Through participation in these programs, survivors become active participants in their own restorative care, rather than passive recipients of doctors' instructions (as survivorship care plans are currently designed). With these skills, survivors are well-equipped to face unforeseen health and psychosocial issues that may arise in the months and years after cancer treatment.

Calls to Action for Patients and Caregivers

» Establish and know your values. You'll be less likely to be blown in the wind, at the mercy of the strongest gust.

» Learn to ask for help.

» Connect with patient advocacy groups to find opportunities to voice your opinion as often and as forcefully as needed. Ask to be included in healthcare board and executive meetings, clinical meetings, and medical conferences. Never give up a chance to provide feedback.

References

Allen, A. (2016). *A tango with cancer: My perilous dance with healthcare and healing.* (n.p.): Oray Publishing.

American College of Surgeons Commission on Cancer. (2016). *Cancer program standards: Ensuring patient-centered care* (2016 Edition). Chicago: Author. Retrieved November 22, 2017, from https://www.facs.org/~/media/files/quality%20programs/cancer/coc/2016%20coc%20standards%20manual_interactive%20pdf.ashx

American Society of Clinical Oncology. (n.d.). Survivorship care plan template. Retrieved March 19, 2017, from http://www.cancer.net/survivorship/follow-care-after-cancer-treatment/asco-cancer-treatment-and-survivorship-care-plans

Bower, J. E., Ganz, P. A., Irwin, M. R., Castellon, S., Arevalo, J., & Cole, S. W. (2013). Cytokine genetic variations and fatigue among patients with breast cancer. *Journal of Clinical Oncology, 31*(13), 1656-1661. doi:10.1200/JCO.2012.46.2143

Brennan, M. E., Gormally, J. F., Butow, P., Boyle, F. M., & Spillane, A. J. (2014). Survivorship care plans in cancer: A systematic review of care plan outcomes. *British Journal of Cancer, 111*(10), 1899-1908. doi:10.1038/bjc.2014.505

Centers for Medicare and Medicaid Services. (2016). Oncology care model. Retrieved December 6, 2017, from https://innovation.cms.gov/initiatives/oncology-care/

Daudt, H., Van Mossel, C., Dennis, D., Leitz, L., Watson, H., & Tanliao, J. (2014). Survivorship care plans: A work in progress. *Current Oncology, 21*(3), e466-e479. doi:10.3747/co.21.1781

Hoffmann T. C., & Del Mar, C. (2017). Clinicians' expectations of the benefits and harms of treatments, screening, and tests: A systematic review. *JAMA Internal Medicine, 177*(3), 407-419. doi:10.1001/jamainternmed.2016.8254

Institute of Medicine and National Research Council. (2005). From cancer patient to cancer survivor: Lost in transition. Washington, D.C.: The National Academies Press. doi:10.17226/11468

Janelsins, M. C., Heckler, C. E., Peppone, L. J., Kamen, C., Mustian, K. M., Mohile, S. G., et al. (2016). Cognitive complaints in survivors of breast cancer after chemotherapy compared with age-matched controls: An analysis from a nationwide, multicenter, prospective longitudinal study. *Journal of Clinical Oncology, 35*(5), 506-514. doi:10.1200/JCO.2016.68.5826

Kesler, S. (2013). Improving cognitive function after cancer. (n.p.): Author.

Livestrong Foundation. (n.d.). Your survivorship care plan. Retrieved March 15, 2017, from https://www.livestrong.org/we-can-help/healthy-living-after-treatment/your-survivorship-care-plan

Llewellyn, A. (2015, October 31). Appropriate utilization of healthcare resources. Retrieved May 20, 2017, from http://www.nursesadvocates.net/2015/10/last-week-i-shared-information-and.html?m=1

Maly, R. C., Liang, L., Liu, Y., Griggs, J. J., & Ganz, P. A. (2016). Randomized controlled trial of survivorship care plans among low-income, predominantly Latina breast cancer survivors. *Journal of Clinical Oncology, 35*(16), 1814-1821. doi:10.1200/JCO.2016.68.9497

Mustian, K. M., Alfano, C. M., Heckler, C., Kleckner, A. S., Kleckner, I. R., Leach, C. R., et al. (2017). Comparison of pharmaceutical, psychological, and exercise treatments for cancer-related fatigue: A meta-analysis. *JAMA Oncology, (3)*7, 961-968. doi:10.1001/jamaoncol.2016.6914

National Cancer Institute. (2017, March 22). Cancer statistics. Retrieved April 30, 2017, from https://www.cancer.gov/about-cancer/understanding/statistics

National Cancer Institute. (2017, March 28). Understanding "chemobrain" and cognitive impairment after cancer treatment. Retrieved May 23, 2017, from http://cancer.gov/about-cancer/treatment/research/understanding-chemobrain

Naughton, M. J., & Weaver, K. E. (2014). Physical and mental health among cancer survivors: Considerations for long-term care and quality of life. *North Carolina Medical Journal, 75*(4), 283-286.

Stordahl, N. (2014). *Getting past the fear: A guide to help you mentally prepare for chemotherapy.* (n.p.): Author.

Chapter Seven: Anchors in the Sand

The rest of us

"Our houses are such unwieldy property, that we are often imprisoned rather than housed in them."

– Henry David Thoreau[1]

This chapter is for everyone who has never had cancer—family, friends, neighbors, or co-workers of people with cancer.

Why a cancer survivorship book for everyone? If you have never had cancer, why should you even think about it?

My response is that there is a massive gap between understanding, knowledge, and action when it comes to health, self-care skills, quality of life, and serious illness. This gap, no doubt, contributes to high U.S. healthcare costs and is detrimental to the quality of care we receive.

In the U.S. we spend nearly twenty percent of our GDP on healthcare, but our outcomes fall far below countries that spend much less. We educate kids on how to succeed in the working world, but we do not teach them how to become healthy adults who can competently navigate the healthcare system and prevent chronic disease.

Current statistics tell us that approximately forty percent of us will have cancer at some point in our lives (National Cancer Institute, 2017). Shouldn't we be preparing people for this prevalent condition?

As it turns out, we do think about cancer often because we are constantly reminded of it— except we think it happens to someone else. Many people do not think about their health until

---

1   Thoreau, 1904, p. 48

a crisis ensues, and we think about death even less. A little education, starting early in life and reinforced over time, could make a big difference when a personal health crisis occurs. It does not take much time, thought, or preparation, but a few key actions can make all the difference.

If you have not thought about cancer before, you ought to start now for the following reasons: 1) at some point in your life, you will have to face cancer, either in yourself or a loved one, 2) because we each play a role in reducing the trauma of cancer, and 3) we can take action to reduce healthcare costs in ways that help ourselves, others, and our economy. In turn, this will improve quality of life for us all.

In this chapter, I describe several of our society's health challenges. Then I discuss how each of us can improve our health, reduce our risk of developing cancer, and improve the likelihood of a better outcome and higher quality of life in survival if we ever do receive a cancer diagnosis.

Challenges in Healthcare

There are more challenges in healthcare than I can address in this book. But despite what seems like a never-ending list below, there is good reason not to get discouraged. We can be proactive in health matters for ourselves and those close to us, on many levels: personally, nationally, and in our communities. Solving matters of social and economic inequality will also be necessary to fully implement solutions, so we serve everyone with cancer, not just those who have access to programs like those in this book.

Lifestyles

We have technological, medical, and scientific advances working to our advantage and steadily increasing our life expectancy, but we could begin to see a reduction in life expectancy due to our lifestyle. In fact, our lifestyle has become a threat to our health. We have too much convenience and too little movement and active engagement with our world. Our communities, for example, contribute to our underactive lifestyle: For many years, commercial and residential areas were separated during planning and development, forcing reliance on cars.

We have become gradually more sedentary in recent decades, increasing our reliance on electronics for work and recreation and partaking in recreational food and alcohol consumption. Nearly half of all people in the U.S. are obese (Centers for Disease Control and Prevention, 2017), and the consequences of that extra weight are diabetes, metabolic disorders, orthopedic problems, cardiovascular disease, and cancer.

Moreover, we martyr ourselves in the service of work. Many people toil to maintain a lifestyle that requires debt or immense stress. While we emphasize achievement and status, too little value is placed on health and quality of life. We should regain awareness of how much we are working and reclaim control of our time for our own energy, quality of life, and longevity.

Medical advances save lives, but medicine is limited in what it can do. While we have increased survival times after cancer, our healthcare costs are steadily increasing and public health outcomes are declining.

<u>Illness-wellness continuum</u>

The illness-wellness continuum[2] provides a visual to understand the concept of health. We are not taught to think about health on a continuum, however. We tend to think of ourselves as either healthy or sick, not about what happens in our bodies on the way to becoming sick.

One's location on the scale is not all-encompassing; it is possible to fall on different locations

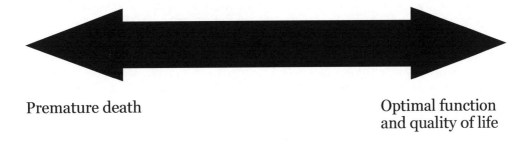

Premature death   Optimal function
                                   and quality of life

along the spectrum with regard to specific aspects of health. For example, one can be extremely physically fit, while also being severely depressed.

We rarely explore the different dimensions of our lives and contemplate their interconnectedness, but our environments and other social factors influence our state of health along this continuum. Health does not exist by itself; it is connected to everything we do.

Interventions must consist of not just information, but skills and action. We often know what we should do, but we have not learned how incorporate healthy behaviors into our lives, while

---

2   The illness-wellness continuum was developed by John W. Travis at the U.S. Public Health Service in 1972. This figure is a simplified version of the continuum designed to give the reader a quick understanding.

navigating the constant temptations, obstacles, setbacks, and relapses that are part of human behavior. Suggestions for introducing these skills are found in the Prevent-Prepare-Prehab program on page A46.

<u>Self-advocacy skills</u>

Self-advocacy skills are needed for good health and optimal outcomes. These skills include critical thinking, self-care skills, willingness to challenge authority, and health, media, consumer, and cancer literacy. These are further described below.

They are not easy skills to attain and hone, but practicing self-advocacy before you must interact with a difficult healthcare system when ill will certainly benefit you.

1. Critical thinking

The *who, what, when, where, how,* and especially *why* questions produce information. Start by routinely asking *why* when being told what to do: Why are you suggesting this course of treatment? Follow up with more questions: What percentage of people are treated successfully? Can I be cured? What are the consequences, risks, and benefits to me? Who will be involved? When can I expect to feel better?

2. Self-care skills

Self-care is most often thought of as proper nutrition and exercise, but taking care of one's mental and emotional health, establishing social supports and financial stability, being free from addiction, and living in a safe environment are at least as important to our health. This requires that we have access to the necessary resources for these self-care actions. Socioeconomic factors can add insurmountable obstacles to the challenges of illness.

3. Challenging authority

Good relationships with healthcare providers are egalitarian, wherein two human beings are exchanging information. Good communication leads to better outcomes.

Unfortunately, many of us have not been taught how to challenge authority. Instead, we are taught to listen to the teacher, obey rules, keep our place, color between the lines, and conform. "Doctor knows best" might be an outdated mindset, but people still do not know how to converse effectively with their doctors or when to seek second opinions. Confidence and courage are the keys to challenging authority, self-advocating, and taking an active role in one's health.

Those raised in families with authoritarian parenting or those who have been victims of abuse may struggle with these skills, but they can be developed in a safe setting with guidance from a trusted professional, such as a mental health worker.

4. Literacy in science, health, media, consumer choices, and technology

In a glut of information, too many people consume advertising and marketing campaigns without questioning their merit, validity, or truth, but a common literacy allows us to meaningfully interact with each other.

Poor literacy in science and health permits myth, mystery, and misinformation about cancer to persist. People are fascinated by cancer, but very little is known among laypeople about what causes cancer, how it develops, its prevalence, how it is treated, why treatments do or do not work, the likelihood of cure or remission, the chance of recurrence, and survival length and quality. This lack of knowledge contributes to a preponderance of fake cures, scams, quackery, and marketing of questionable therapies that can make treatment choices even more confusing.

Schattner (2017) clarifies a number of issues in current media reporting on cancer that can influence public health outcomes. The Cancer Harbors module titled "About Online and Printed Information" (found at https://cancerharbors.com/table-of-contents-cancer-harbors/) teaches skills and provides resources for discerning factual and scientifically accurate information.

5. Cancer literacy

It seems that every day I hear someone say, "I don't know how I got cancer! I ate right, exercised, managed my stress, never smoked, had no family history…"

Many people mistakenly think they are immune to cancer if they lead the right lifestyle, but this is just an illusion of control. We can manage what we put in our mouths or do to our bodies, but we are all still made of cells. Cells have DNA, and DNA can mutate.

A basic healthcare education curriculum in primary schools is needed. People need to know a few basic facts—that not all cancers are the same, that every cancer acts differently, and that all patients are treated differently. Everyone should have a basic understanding of the physiology of the human body (how it works), to make it easier to understand cancer pathophysiology (the impact of cancer on the body).

No two people will have the same cancer experience. Comparing one person's experience to another's will almost certainly be inaccurate. For this reason, avoid giving advice to someone with cancer based on your knowledge of your own or someone else's experience. Support them with your knowledge, but leave treatment decisions to the patient and his or her doctor.

Further, the more we know about cancer, the better we can support loved ones and acquaintances with cancer. There are more ways to offer support than telling them to fight. Cheerleading and battle cries may not be what they need to hear at that moment.

The Cancer Harbors website contains suggestions for how to support people with cancer (https://cancerharbors.com/anatomy/). It also contains modules to help you acquire the self-advocacy skills described above (https://cancerharbors.com/table-of-contents-cancer-harbors/). These modules are listed on the following page.

Fear and denial around mortality

Very few people get what they hope for: a painless, quick death in their sleep. For most people, it is a slow, gradual decline marked by suffering. Cancer awakens our fears of pain, death, and losing control. But recognizing our mortality helps us savor our time and consider our values. (See the Values Exercise on page A8 for strategies to consciously consider your values around health and quality of life.)

We spend most of our healthcare dollars on end-of-life care in hospitals, with complex and expensive interventions that often do not yield quality survival time. If we could accept that we do not have to do everything possible to save a dying person's life, we may find that cancer patients have higher quality of life while they remain with us. When someone dies from cancer, it is not shameful, and they have not failed—and neither has their doctor.

Understanding palliative care

Palliative care is managing symptoms and providing comfort to improve quality of life, while supporting the patient and his or her family. Hospice care is palliative care at the end of life. Referring a patient to palliative care, and understanding the difference between palliative and hospice care, is one of the most important ways a doctor can support the patient's quality of life needs.

Because of palliative care's association with death, it is now referred to by many healthcare organizations as supportive care. I believe a better approach is to embrace palliative care as

Cancer Harbors modules for caregivers and people without cancer

Exercise vs. physical activity:
Understanding the difference

Healthy foods vs. healthy diet

Indoor restorative environments

Outdoor restorative environments

A self-care exercise

Taking responsibility for your ongoing
health

Prevention, risk & cause

Lifelong learning

Supplements, diets & fads

Caloric intake, food choices, and eating at
home; Actions to take/checklist

Weight loss, abdominal fat, emotions,
stress and sleep

Balancing energy

Diaphragmatic breathing

Journaling and expressive therapies

Time & energy conservation

Self-advocacy in communicating with
doctors about symptoms, side effects, and
pain

Interpreting research studies reported in
the media

Online & printed information for health
consumers

Using social media & Tweetchats for
information & support

---

acceptable in all circumstances, to accept and embrace our mortality, and to provide humane healthcare throughout the lifespan and regardless of where we fall on the illness-wellness continuum.

Inaction

At the time of publishing this book, we do not know what the future holds for healthcare legislation or the Affordable Care Act. But what we need is a system that removes, or at least controls, the influence of powerful entities like pharmaceutical companies, insurance companies, and the hospital industry. We need a healthcare system that serves all citizens with equitable healthcare services and that is focused on addressing the social issues that lead to poor population health, such as poverty and wealth inequality.

Regardless of where you stand on the political spectrum, there are problems with the healthcare system, most notably related to lack of transparency. There is documented evidence of greed and price gouging—both in healthcare facilities (Xu et al., 2017) and by drug companies, such as the recent high-profile Daraprim® and Epi-Pen® scandals.

Voicing your opinion to your elected representatives and putting pressure on those responsible is essential. You and your family will benefit from making the system more equitable. You will feel great pride and see results if you act on issues that are important to you.

Inability to ask for help

A common characteristic among many of my clients is an inability to ask for help. For some people, it truly is daunting to ask for help. Even more difficult is learning to recognize when you need help. Mental health support is a perfect example: The stigma associated with mental illness keeps far too many people from getting the help they need to cope with life, let alone the stress of cancer.

Not wanting to be seen as weak or needy is a product of the socially stigmatizing "pull yourself up by your bootstraps" mentality so prevalent in our society. But when people's emotional or basic physical needs are chronically unmet, whether during childhood or adulthood, they may express their needs in the form of dependence on healthcare resources—that is, they may actually get sick more often.

This "bootstraps" mentality is often accompanied by a lack of empathy and victim-blaming, even in some healthcare circles. For example, patients who frequently seek healthcare have been referred to as "frequent flyers," a subtly disparaging term.

Lack of understanding of the healthcare industry

Healthcare is big business, and most people do not give it much thought until they interact with it. Big business relies on big marketing campaigns, and they can be extremely misleading but persuasive. Lomangino (2017) identifies a four-step process for misleading consumers about health news and inconclusive research findings, by convincing viewers that a breakthrough in treatment is available and can be attributed to an organization or its medical staff.

One needed change nearly everyone agrees on is cost reduction. Healthcare costs are not transparent, but we do know we are not getting a good value for our healthcare dollars spent, when we compare our statistics to those of other industrialized nations.

Big business healthcare is highly data-driven. Administrators of big healthcare systems are consumed with evaluating data on cost, efficiency, productivity, and outcomes. This has driven up healthcare administrative costs astronomically. It remains to be seen whether these administrative expenditures will pay off in terms of safety, quality, and outcomes for patients.

Lack of understanding of healthcare providers' roles

Many patients have limited understanding of healthcare providers' roles, their limits, and who can fill in the gaps. Nurses, medical assistants, nurse practitioners, physician assistants, social workers, and administrative staff all work in oncology practices, along with other professionals. (The roles of various healthcare staff are explained in the appendix on page A39.)

It is helpful to understand the roles and responsibilities of the various providers you see. Healthcare appointments are short, and doctors have limited time to address complicated questions. Everything you can do to simplify the process will help you make the most of your appointment. To start, keep track of your medications and health history, and bring updated health records.

Learn what healthcare workers outside your physician's office, such as pharmacists, care coordinators, and dietitians, can do for you, and do not be afraid to ask for referrals.

Uncertainty about how to support someone with cancer

It can be difficult to know what to say and do for someone who has recently been diagnosed with cancer. Even if you are a skilled and tactful communicator, you may experience uncomfortable conversations. This is because we often still associate cancer with death. Reminding yourself that many people recover from cancer, and that they may need your help, can help you thoughtfully extend support.

When trying to support someone who has cancer, do not speculate on why they got it, and instead focus on what you can do for them. There are two areas people tend to need help most: first, managing the sheer number of appointments, and second, the work of recovery after treatment.

Being a cancer patient is a full-time job. There are procedures, scans, tests, labs, doctor visits, surgeries, treatment visits, follow-up visits, and more, none of which ever seem to be convenient or at the same time or place. Anything you can do to save them time and energy—cooking, laundry, cleaning, pet care, yard work, or grocery shopping, for example—will be appreciated.

After treatment ends, there are fewer appointments, but there is anxiety and lingering fatigue. Survivors have difficulty trusting their body, and they may experience holdover symptoms from treatment that make it difficult to return to normal activities or a full schedule. Do not disappear; the person still needs you.

The Cancer Harbors page titled, "How to Help the Person in Your Life with Cancer" (https://cancerharbors.com/anatomy/) provides guidelines on what to do and what not to do when someone you know has been diagnosed. Learn as much as you can so you can offer good support. Don't let emotion take over where realistic help, support, recovery, healing, and learning need to be. You can be an anchor without sinking the ship.

Caregivers

No one expects to become a caregiver any more than they expect to become a patient, and our healthcare system supports caregivers even less. Despite much jargon about patient- and family-centered care, we do not do this well in practice. Only hospice and palliative care truly work this concept into their philosophies and practice. The rest of our healthcare system relies on at least half a trillion dollars in uncompensated care each year from caregivers (AARP, 2016).

Caregivers are, out of necessity and regardless of preparedness, the primary advocates for patients. They need at least as much education as the patient about the disease, its treatment, how to care for the patient, and how to help the patient recover. Lacking a medical or nursing background, caregivers can become lost. They need basic guidance on when to call the doctor as opposed to go to the ER, or how to address common problems such as fever, nausea, pain, and fatigue. The caregiver must be included in all conversations from the beginning to post-treatment to address lingering concerns, follow-up care, and functioning.

Thus far, I have described numerous challenges in cancer care. Taken together, they may seem overwhelming. But let's chip away at them, in pieces. Let's put our efforts into impacting people's lives on a small scale, by managing resources wisely and with compassion. Then we can begin to close the gaps in care.

Whether you do this on a personal, community-wide, or national level is your choice, based on where you feel you can make the most difference with your skills and resources. Below are several solutions, so you can start working today.

Solutions

The following are several ideas for improvements to our current approach to cancer. More specific guidelines for building skills and action are included in the appendix. The following solutions apply to everyone, regardless of your role in or around healthcare, or your cancer or health status.

1. Creativity, authenticity, resourcefulness, and empathy

We must be creative and resourceful in our approaches to multifaceted problems. Changes to cancer care will take a lot of effort, and the people best-equipped to address needed change are those who have been through it themselves. Listen to people who have had cancer, as they provide the best support for other people with cancer. Doctors and nurses who have not experienced cancer themselves should respect this, as well.

Survivors play a key role in educating the public, and their perspectives are important to ongoing efforts to improve care on the part of researchers, administrators, and healthcare providers. But everyone, regardless of their relationship to cancer, is a stakeholder in cancer survivorship and can take an active role in advocating for responsible policy and legislation around healthcare. Cultivate empathy by appealing to the human qualities of leaders and elected officials.

We are all swimming in the same ocean. The person next to you is made from the same cells that you are, but with his or her own unique genetic code. Each of us will be sick and need to rely on others for help at some point in our lives. Everyone has experienced pain or trauma of some sort. If you can identify with the struggle of not having control and trying to recover from that frightening experience, you can empathize with the experience of having cancer.

Offer support when you can, but do not assume you know what another person is experiencing or that they feel the way you do. What one person can handle well may be a crisis for the next, depending on their own coping resources, experience, or perception. Cancer requires a support network, but not everyone is the right support person for someone else. Don't take it personally. Instead, be authentic, and offer help and support graciously.

Simply put, be kind and don't expect too much from cancer survivors. Healing takes time and occurs on many levels. This is especially important for employers, coworkers, friends, and family to remember.

2. **Learn**

The Cancer Harbors modules on health literacy teach skills for understanding media reports on cancer research and further becoming an informed consumer of products, services, and information.

Start by passing over the clickbait articles that grab your attention while you surf online. At best, they discourage deep thought; at worst, they perpetuate inaccurate myths and convince readers to make poor health decisions. Practice building a longer attention span by reading scientific articles that require extended focus, even taking notes to stay on track.

Learn about the scientific method and why you should not change your behavior based on the results of one study. When reading about cancer studies in the media, be on the lookout for details about the research method, such as sample size, time frame, details about the subjects, and whether it was randomized or non-randomized.

Learn also about risk, the likelihood of an event occurring in the general population, and the likelihood of that event happening to you. Doctors often talk in terms of risk, but it is important to know your own risk before making medical decisions that could affect your future. (Refer to the Cancer Harbors module, "Prevention, Risk & Cause" at https://cancerharbors.com/table-of-contents-cancer-harbors/.)

Learn about cancer. Assume it will happen to you or someone close to you. But that does not mean you should not do everything in your power to avoid it. Accepting the realities of cancer means you can prepare mentally, emotionally, socially, and legally for serious illness.

Life is not over for someone with advanced cancer, but people with Stage IV cancer often feel forgotten, and laypeople and healthcare providers both should not dismiss their survivorship needs. Their concerns are likely not only with end-of-life planning, and they deserve all the opportunities and options of comprehensive healthcare.

3. **Plan—even before you need it**

The Prevent-Prepare-Prehab program (page A46) explains what informed citizens should know to navigate the healthcare system during a serious illness. Taking an active role in planning for unexpected events will save you and your family a lot of worry, stress, and anxiety.

Build your network and rally your resources before a crisis. It is one of the most valuable preparations you can make right now. It is helpful to spread your requests for help around, to avoid overburdening a primary caregiver, who will have numerous responsibilities in your care.

Think about who you will be able to rely on. Relatives, friends, coworkers, or neighbors? Who are your best resources for the myriad tasks you will need help with, such as cooking, cleaning, yard work, or driving to appointments? Who is strong enough to do the heavy lifting, literally and figuratively? Who can attend appointments with you as an advocate, taking notes and asking questions on your behalf?

Prepare a broad list of questions you might ask in the event of a cancer (or other illness) diagnosis. You do not need a crystal ball to anticipate questions. Simply start by thinking about illnesses that have befallen your own family members and others you know. Keep the list at your disposal, and take it with you to healthcare appointments, even routine doctor visits. Remember that *why* is the most important question you can ask when discussing healthcare options.

(Questions to ask upon diagnosis with cancer are provided on page 75, so you may wish to start there. The Cancer Harbors modules on self-advocacy, found at https://cancerharbors. com/table-of-contents-cancer-harbors/, will also help you build skills around healthcare interactions.)

Prepare and discuss your advance directives with those closest to you, even if you are young, healthy, and feel no expectation of cancer or illness. Keep a copy of your advance directives in your medical record, and discuss them with your primary care provider. You can update, change, or revoke them at any time. It is recommended to update them regularly, especially after important life events.

Put yourself in control, and set yourself up for optimal care now. The Prevent-Prepare-Prehab program goes into more detail about these steps.

4. Take an active role in your own health

First, take care of your health issues now. The fewer unresolved health problems you have going into a serious illness, the less complicated your treatment will be. For example, if you are struggling with untreated depression or anxiety, communicate your concerns to your physician now. Learn about your condition and what treatment will work best.

Complicating the most serious, and not to mention expensive, health problems—mental illness, substance abuse, and chronic disease—is lack of communication with one's healthcare provider. By communicating early and often, you will receive the education and treatment you need for these conditions before they become difficult to control.

Next, challenge yourself both physically and mentally. If you are using an electronic gadget, set the timer to remind yourself it is time to take a break and do something physical. In my opinion, all devices should flash periodically with the message, "Put me down and move!" Look for opportunities for physical activity. It can be as simple as taking a walk around the field while you are waiting to pick up your child from soccer practice.

The American College of Sports Medicine currently provides recommendations for the minimum amount of physical activity to achieve health benefits. They recommend either 30 minutes a day, 5 times a week, of moderate physical activity such as walking; or 20 minutes, 3 days a week, of vigorous physical activity (Garber et al., 2011).

Many people exercise far below the level of intensity necessary to reap the benefits, however. Tracking devices to count steps per day can raise your awareness of the duration of activity needed to meet these basic health recommendations, but they will not ensure you are working hard enough. Newer tracking devices monitor the intensity of your activity so you can achieve greater health benefits.

5. Don't just do; enjoy

Slow down, and engage in physical, emotional, and spiritual renewal processes. Instead of doing and achieving all the time, try to simply be, soak it all in, and take pleasure in small, simple things. Put your electronic gadgets away, clear your mind, then explore, re-evaluate, make decisions, and rebuild when you are refreshed and ready. Good health requires active thought about what we do with our time, and it ultimately impacts the quality of our lives.

The FIERCE program through Cancer Harbors allows clients to explore mind-body therapies that reduce stress, manage anxiety, and improve fitness, as well as establishing social connections and finding social support among other survivors. Recreational pursuits and fun are part of a high-quality life.

The Cancer Harbors module on expressive therapies can guide you in creative pursuits, such as art, music, or writing. The restorative environments modules help you create restorative spaces that enhance healing, whether in the home, workplace, or peaceful settings outdoors.

(The modules can be found at https://cancerharbors.com/table-of-contents-cancer-harbors/.) Do not underestimate the power of your surroundings to influence your healing. People have shorter surgical recovery times when their hospital room has a view of nature as opposed to a wall (Ulrich, 1984).

Moving Forward

Merely by living your life, you have acquired countless skills and resources that you can rely on to manage your health. Maintain awareness of the many factors that affect your health, reach out for help when you need it, and offer support to others when you can. Your environment, social network, family, occupation, recreational pursuits, unaddressed fears, beliefs, background, and support systems are important.

With the help of Cancer Harbors materials, such as the Prevent-Prepare-Prehab contents (page A46) and self-advocacy modules (https://cancerharbors.com/table-of-contents-cancer-harbors/), I recommend you fill your gaps in preparation, find appropriate resources, and build more skills to help yourself and others.

Read about the Cancer Harbors program in its abbreviated form in the appendix, or visit the Cancer Harbors website to view the entire program. You can also access the video coaching component of the program there.

Taking responsibility for your own health as an individual is important, but let's take it further. Each of us plays an important role in our collective public health. My dream, as idealistic as it may sound, is that we all feel a duty to become educated about our health, with the goal of sustaining a healthcare system that truly serves every one of us.

Calls to Action for the Rest of Us

» Don't live in denial of your own fallibility. Stop pretending you will never have to deal with a serious illness and death.

» Take responsibility for your entire life, and that includes your death. Once you've made your plans, you can sit back and enjoy living.

» Teach yourself to have a longer attention span. Read long articles, taking notes to stay on track. Look up terms you don't understand. Ask why, often. Find people to explain confusing concepts to you.

» Vote and have a voice in the political process, even if it is distasteful to you. We cannot afford apathy; we must speak out when we perceive injustice. This is one way to give back to your fellow human beings, your community, your country, and the world.

References

Centers for Disease Control and Prevention. (2017, August 29). Obesity facts. Retrieved October 20, 2017, from https://www.cdc.gov/obesity/data/adult.html

Garber, C. E., Blissmer, B., Deschenes, M. R., Franklin, B. A., Lamonte, M. J., Lee, I. M., et al. (2011). American College of Sports Medicine position stand. Quantity and quality of exercise for developing and maintaining cardiorespiratory, musculoskeletal, and neuromotor fitness in apparently healthy adults: Guidance for prescribing exercise. *Medicine & Science in Sports & Exercise, 43*(7), 1334-1359. doi:10.1249/MSS.0b013e318213fefb

Jenkins, J. A. (2016, November 14). Caregiving costly to family caregivers. Retrieved May 23, 2017, from http://www.aarp.org/home-family/caregiving/info-2016/caregiving-costly-to-family-caregivers-jj.html

Lomangino, K. (2017, May 26). We are in a crisis of crap health news—this week's reporting shows why. *Health News Review*. Retrieved May 30, 2017, from https://www.healthnewsreview.org/2017/05/we-are-in-a-crisis-of-crap-health-news-this-weeks-reporting-shows-why/

National Cancer Institute. (2017, March 22). Cancer statistics. Retrieved April 30, 2017, from https://www.cancer.gov/about-cancer/understanding/statistics

Schattner, E. (2017, August 31). Can cancer truths be told? Challenges for medical journalism. *ASCO Current Insights in Oncology*. Retrieved September 20, 2017, from https://connection.asco.org/magazine/current-controversies-oncology/excerpt-can-cancer-truths-be-told

Thoreau, H. D. (1904). *Walden*. London: George Routledge & Sons. Retrieved November 17, 2017, from https://books.google.com/books?id=YXJbAAAAMAAJ&printsec=frontcover#v=onepage&q&f=false

Ulrich, R. S. (1984). View through a window may influence recovery from surgery. *Science, 224*(4647), 420-421.

Xu, T., Park, A., Bai, G., Joo, S., Hutfless, S. M., Mehta, A., et al. (2017). Variation in emergency department vs internal medicine excess charges in the United States. *JAMA Internal Medicine, 177*(8), 1139-1145. doi:10.1001/jamainternmed.2017.1598

Chapter Eight: Setting Sail

Moving forward

"We should take care not to make the intellect our God; it has, of course, powerful muscles, but no personality."

– Albert Einstein[1]

I stated several goals at the beginning of this book—to inspire action and advocacy and to empower patients, physicians, nurses, and other stakeholders to self-advocate. I illuminated what happens behind the scenes in healthcare and how treatment of cancer can bring about more trauma than necessary.

My intention is that after reading this book, you will begin to build the necessary skills:

» As a patient or potential patient, to take control of your own health, as you cannot rely on the healthcare industry to do it for you.

» As a healthcare professional, to take control of your everyday practice, as you must demand freedom, time, and a reasonable workload to be able to care for patients' needs as well as your own, to get involved in your community, and to connect with providers of complementary services outside your organization.

» As a human being, foremost, to stop *doing* for a moment, so you can think and define your values and be sure you are acting in accordance with those values. When you do that, you will be stronger in demanding what you need and achieving what you desire in life.

We gain nothing by continuing down the current path. Instead, let's be generous with the resources and tools we have at our disposal. Let's foster creativity, authenticity, resourcefulness,

---

1 Rowe & Schulmann, 2007, p. 322

and empathy. Let's put our resources in the right places, come together, and make it work.

Many people are already doing this work and building communities around it. Community programs in the nonprofit and for-profit sectors help patients and contribute resources for those in need. Programs similar to FIERCE and Cancer Harbors, which are detailed throughout the book and in the appendix, can be found throughout the country.

We must leave our silos and talk to each other in citizen discussion groups that represent all stakeholders. We have a growing number of older citizens who have the interest and time to devote to leading such efforts. Why not have community-based senior "health corps" tasked with bringing together people of all ages and roles?

We on the front lines—physicians, nurses, and professional healthcare workers—can use our voices and influence to make change. We may encounter discomfort as we confront the dysfunctional system we have enabled with our silence, complacency, and apathy. Healthcare leaders must learn what is truly valuable—that is, care that contributes to patients' quality of life—and put resources exclusively into the services that deliver this value. Hundreds of thousands of nurses are disillusioned with nursing but would welcome opportunities to use their knowledge, skills, and wisdom in the true service of patient outcomes and quality of life.

Citizens—including cancer patients, survivors, caregivers, family, and friends of those with cancer, and even those who have never had cancer—play a role. Take five or ten minutes per day, or even per week, to become more informed and speak out on issues that affect you. Write letters to your representatives. Read the most factual, unbiased sources of news and information you can find.

Action is required. If we think of the healthcare system as a metaphor for health, we are looking at a system made chronically ill by an under-informed, distracted, and sedentary public. We need to move—it does not take much, but each of us needs to do our part. What we do or don't do ultimately affects everyone else. When someone has cancer, we all are affected.

A good start is to examine our values with regard to our health and quality of life. The Values Exercise (page A8) is intended for everyone, regardless of cancer status or role in healthcare.

My takeaway message to fellow healthcare providers is this: Let's venture beyond merely treating disease. We must transcend the survivorship care plan to reduce the risk of cancer recurrence, to help patients enjoy better health and quality of life, and to truly heal patients whose diseases have been treated.

Let's remember that survivorship does not exist in a clinic; it is everyday life for people who have had cancer. Therefore, instead of instructing patients, we should assess their interests and values. Even patients who show normal labs and are breathing, talking, and walking in their office visits may be experiencing issues with their everyday functions. Simply allowing patients to report issues at their own convenience—rather than the convenience of healthcare providers—improves health-related quality of life (Basch et al., 2015).

Cancer Harbors and other similar programs provide expert support and guidance that cancer survivors seek, especially after treatment. Referrals to less-clinical community resources help survivors return to a more normal lifestyle. Referrals are tailored to individual needs, meaning they bridge life as a "cancer patient" with life as a "survivor."

In my own practice, I begin with a client assessment. I ask intake questions about health behaviors and their comfort with those behaviors. I assess clients' personal strengths and deficits, their interest in health, their self-efficacy, and how they learn. This allows me to direct them to resources of interest to them. They will be more likely to use information that fits their lifestyle.

This process takes time, and it requires skill, listening, and thought from both the client and the provider. Between the initial meeting and assessment, check-ins, and follow-up at the end, I spend six months getting to know my clients well enough to refer them to other services. My clients spend equal time sharing their experiences with me.

Programs like Cancer Harbors become demonstrably worthwhile for patients when you consider that eight hours of professional time can spare patients countless hours of lost time, frustration, and potentially missing out on needed services. What's more, they receive support along the way. Further research is needed on these programs' effects on survivorship outcomes, quality of life, and healthcare costs.

Changing the healthcare culture will take time. Presently, the healthcare system so often misses the positive contributions of interdisciplinary treatments and therapies. It will take time for research trials to be funded and conducted, for the results to be reviewed and published, and for changes to be made to healthcare practices. This culture shift will be a long haul. Let us not forget that while we are waiting for change, we must act to prevent suffering now.

* * *

My takeaway message to my fellow citizens is this: Let's rejuvenate a spirit of caring for ourselves and each other. Let's make a wide array of treatments and therapies available, accessible, and affordable for everyone, so we all benefit from greater health and quality of life.

This will require action from all of us. This is what it will take to restore our physical, mental, and spiritual health. Together we have the opportunity to acknowledge our vulnerability to illness and improve our shared quality of life.

Be creative. Find a way to do something different, try something that no one else has tried, or do it with a new twist. Challenge mediocrity and risk-aversion.

Be authentic. Tell your story, whether you're a patient, a healthcare worker, or a caregiver. Share your experiences and what you have learned.

Be resourceful. Take an inventory of what you have—tools, skills, knowledge, and most important, people—and put them to work without reinventing the wheel. Do the best you can with what you already have.

Have empathy. Listen and try to relate to the human experience you share with others.

Begin Now: Resources Are at Your Fingertips

The appendix that follows is comprised of programs for cancer survivors. I developed these programs, and they are currently in use in my own community. I include a proposed curriculum for educating the public. I also explain the theoretical basis for these programs in social-cognitive models of health behavior.

> » The FIERCE program is an active support program for cancer survivors to increase enjoyment of physical activity and movement for restoring health and well-being.

> » The Cancer Harbors program is a six-month program for skill-based learning on restoring quality of life for cancer survivors.

> » The Prevent-Prepare-Prehab curriculum teaches the public how to be more informed about healthcare and to advocate for themselves and their loved ones in the event of a diagnosis of cancer or other serious illness.

> » I also include a short section on athletes with cancer. Working with a healthcare system that is generally accustomed to a less-fit population can be a challenge for athletes, especially for those who wish to expedite a return to the sport they love.

I offer the Cancer Harbors service via online videoconferencing sessions, along with distribution of the remaining Cancer Harbors modules according to individual client needs. I offer individual and group coaching services. To find out more about these services and their availability, please visit the Cancer Harbors website at https://cancerharbors.com/.

I provide consulting services for organizations wishing to incorporate the FIERCE or Cancer Harbors models into their facilities. More information is available at the Cancer Harbors website. I encourage ambitious, disruptive, and groundbreaking researchers to pursue studies of these programs to examine their benefits to cancer survivors in terms of outcomes, quality of life, and costs.

We're all in the boat. Now we must raise our anchors, steer toward calmer waters, and find a tailwind. I hope you'll sail with me.

References

Basch, E., Deal, A. M., Kris, M. G., Scher, H. I., Hudis, C. A., Sabbatini, P., et al. (2016). Symptom monitoring with patient-reported outcomes during routine cancer treatment: A randomized controlled trial. *Journal of Clinical Oncology, 34*(6), 557-565. doi:10.1200/JCO.2015.63.0830

Rowe, D. E., & Schulmann, R. (Eds.). (2007). *Einstein on politics: His private thoughts and public stands on nationalism, Zionism, war, peace, and the bomb.* Princeton, New Jersey: Princeton University Press. Retrieved November 17, 2017, from https://books.google.com/books?id=AIHgK-p6mhgC&printsec=frontcover#v=onepage&q&f=false

Final Words

I hope you have found *Navigating the C: A Nurse Charts the Course for Cancer Survivorship Care* to be insightful and helpful in preparing for, recovering from, or living with cancer, or in treating and caring for someone with cancer. Cancer encompasses such a wide range of information, and our body of knowledge about cancer changes quickly, so there is much I could not include in this book. The Cancer Harbors modules at https://cancerharbors.com/table-of-contents-cancer-harbors/ will be updated as new information becomes available.

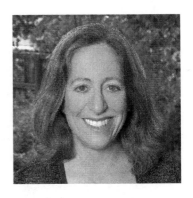

If you would like to contact me directly, please feel free to e-mail me at info@cancerharbors.com.

Alene Nitzky, Ph.D., RN, OCN
Cancer Harbors
www.cancerharbors.com

Appendix

Introduction

Why do you need the Cancer Harbors and FIERCE programs as a healthcare consumer?

If you want to get the best care from your doctor and other healthcare providers, you must do your part to be prepared, ask appropriate questions, and do your own research and footwork. Cancer Harbors and FIERCE help you build your knowledge and skills around self-care. You can assist your doctors in providing excellent healthcare by being an informed patient who takes an active role in your own care. Cancer Harbors is a complement to a doctor's care, not a substitute.

There are many concerns and topics around cancer care that doctors do not have time to discuss with their patients. It's not because they are trying to hide anything from you. They might not be aware of your needs, they might not have the skills to address the specific topics, or they might not know of someone who offers complementary health services. They may simply not have time in their busy days to do the research themselves. Doctors often have difficulty keeping up with the demands of their specialty. This is especially true for oncologists, with the avalanche of new information and research on cancer that comes out every day. This is why it is up to you, the patient, to take an active role if you want to achieve your best possible health.

Just because your doctor does not discuss certain topics with you, it does not mean your concerns are not important. Doctors cannot get a snapshot of what you are experiencing every day unless you are very organized, concise, and descriptive in your discussions with them. When you are fatigued, distracted, or busy, it can be very difficult to provide every pertinent detail in the short period in the doctor's office.

Your doctors plan and prescribe cancer treatments, but they usually have not experienced cancer themselves. They cannot feel what you are experiencing in your own body. Since doctors do not go through everyday life in your shoes, they have no idea how you are affected on a day-to-day, moment-to-moment basis.

If your doctor does talk about the following topics and refers you to professionals who can help you address or resolve them, you have an exceptional doctor! If your doctor or doctors are in the exceptional group, thank them for it.

The following are areas in which Cancer Harbors can help you build knowledge and skills and find resources.

» The importance of physical activity and finding guidance and support in sticking to a regular routine that is challenging enough to provide health benefits. FIERCE provides such guidance.

» Mental health needs beyond prescription medications such as antidepressants. Counseling and psychological and emotional support are very important.

» Weighing the risks and benefits of various therapies, including discussing potential side effects and their effects on quality of life.

» Minimizing the risk of recurrence of your cancer and developing a contingency plan.

» Changes in your body image, appearance, and functional abilities at home, work, and leisure.

» Effects of treatment and the experience of cancer on everyday life.

» Finding online information that is accurate and evidence-based.

» Complementary therapies and their availability in the community.

» Prehabilitation and how to prepare yourself for future interventions or surgeries.

» Stressors on you and your family, including finances and health.

» Contributors to fatigue like endocrine disorders or nutritional deficiencies.

» The long-term effects of cancer treatment and how to cope with them.

» Dental considerations: how your teeth, jaw, and mouth may be affected by chemotherapy and radiation, and the long-term effects on your dental health.

» Incontinence, erectile dysfunction, sexual dysfunction, and intimacy difficulties.

» Encouraging you to get second and third opinions if you have an advanced stage of cancer, a rare form of cancer, or are running out of treatment options.

» Using palliative care (also called supportive care) to relieve symptoms and improve quality of life regardless of your prognosis. (Even early stage cancer patients with an excellent likelihood of long-term survival without recurrence can benefit from supportive care during treatment.)

» End-of-life considerations when warranted, and encouraging conversation around advance directives for everyone.

Disclaimer

Cancer Harbors®, FIERCE: Functional & Fit, Independent, Energized, Restored, Confident, & Empowered®, and Sunspirit Wellness Services, LLC, do not provide medical advice or nursing care, and do not prescribe medications, supplements, or products, or diagnose, treat, or cure any condition or illness. The information in the videos, online, and in printed and downloadable materials is not medical advice nor nursing care, and is not a substitute for, and should not be construed as, medical advice or nursing care. For medical advice, consult a licensed physician.

Not all exercise is suitable for everyone. Before attempting any new exercise, flexibility, strength, and overall health must be considered to determine if a specific exercise is appropriate for you. Any exercise is inherently dangerous and can result in personal injury. Any injury sustained from proper or improper use of the exercises in this book and linked video materials is solely the responsibility of the exerciser. Cancer Harbors®, FIERCE: Functional & Fit, Independent, Energized, Restored, Confident, & Empowered®, and Sunspirit Wellness Services, LLC, and their staff, representatives, successors, and assigns disclaim any liability from injury sustained from the use of the exercises in this book and linked video materials and suggest that you consult your physician before attempting any exercise or exercise program.

As with any exercise program, if at any point during your workout, you begin to feel dizzy, faint, lightheaded, or have physical discomfort, you should stop immediately. You are responsible for exercising within your limits and seeking medical advice and attention as appropriate. The content in this book and linked video materials and the exercise tips and instructions are not a substitute for medical advice. If you are concerned about whether the exercises in this or any exercise program are right for you, do not do them until you have received clearance from your physician.

Appendix Contents

The Theoretical Basis for the Programs

I want to briefly explain the theoretical underpinnings for the following programs. My academic background combines physiological health benefits and social/behavioral science as they both apply to recreation and activities that improve quality of life. Theories of health behavior and behavior change, motivation, and learning have fed the development of these programs.

Basic research is driven by theory, and it allows us to carry our body of understanding forward as we make scientific discoveries and build a body of evidence to influence clinical and community practice.

The FIERCE: Functional & Fit, Independent, Energized, Restored, Confident, & Empowered® program builds physical activity into a lifestyle, encourages and supports its maintenance through social networking and regular meetings with a qualified instructor and coach, overcomes barriers by providing a non-competitive, non-intimidating, and convenient setting, and includes regular follow-up communication.

The Cancer Harbors® program builds skills in self-care, self-advocacy, and health behaviors through educational materials that users can choose based on their individual preferences, at their own pace and at their own convenience, with a minimal commitment of time over a six-month period. Cancer Harbors also provides guided coaching by a professional health coach to build self-efficacy around these skills.

The following theories have influenced my work:

The Health Belief Model (Rosenstock, 1974) suggests that health behavior depends upon self-perception of the severity of an illness and susceptibility to that illness, and weighing the barriers against the benefits of taking action to change behavior.

Learning theories, such as the Social Learning Theory (Bandura, 1977), use social and cognitive approaches to propose that learning behavior occurs through human responses via teaching, reinforcement, practice, observation, and modeling the behavior.

Self-efficacy is an important construct in all of these theories. I define self-efficacy as a person's confidence in their own ability to perform a behavior, and it is specific to a situation. The more self-efficacy a person has in a particular behavior, the more likely he or she is to perform it successfully.

The Transtheoretical Model (Stages of Change) by Prochaska and DiClemente (1983) explains readiness for health behavior change by the cognitive and behavioral processes by which a person changes their behavior. Decisions are made by weighing pros and cons at each individual stage, and self-efficacy contributes to the readiness for change, from the pre-contemplation, contemplation, and preparation stages, through action, maintenance, and termination (success) stages of the change process.

Ecological Approaches explain health behavior as being determined by interpersonal, intrapersonal, public policy, community, and institutional factors (McLeroy, Steckler, & Bibeau, 1988).

Regarding these theoretical approaches, the programs here are based in learning new behaviors and skills through group and individual experiences in the community, as well as building self-efficacy around these skills through social support, guidance, and coaching by a qualified instructor.

The programs provide opportunities to reduce the risk of cancer development and recurrence via health behavior modification, with periodic follow-ups for relapse prevention, to maintain the healthy behavior changes.

References

Bandura, A. (1977). Self-efficacy: Toward a unifying theory of behavioral change. *Psychological Review, 84*(2), 191-215.

McLeroy, K. R., Steckler, A., & Bibeau, D. (1988). The social ecology of health promotion interventions. *Health Education Quarterly, 15*, 351-377.

Prochaska, J. O., & DiClemente, C. C. (1983). Stages and processes of self-change of smoking: Toward an integrative model of change. *Journal of Consulting and Clinical Psychology, 51*(3), 390-395.

Rosenstock, I. (1974). Historical origins of the health belief model. *Health Education Monographs, 2*(4): 328-335. doi:10.1177/109019817400200403

Values Exercise

The Values Exercise provides an opportunity to consciously consider your values around health and quality of life. It will guide you in setting priorities and aligning your behaviors with what is most important to you. Take time to answer the following questions, independent of anything you have learned in the past or what someone else has told you. If you have never been diagnosed with cancer, skip questions 6 & 7.

1   How do you define health for yourself?

2   How do you define living and quality of life?

3   How well and to what extent are you living up to each of those definitions now?

4   If you are not living up to your definitions, what do you need to do and what resources do you need to do it?

5   Do you need to change your plans or your expectations of yourself or others to achieve the health and quality of life you want? If so, how will you do that?

6   Of everything that you have gone through since your cancer diagnosis, what would you have liked to know beforehand, and what information would have helped you cope, have a better experience, make things go smoothly, or avoid trauma?

7   Have your definitions of health and quality of life changed since your diagnosis? If so, how?

Alene Nitzky

FIERCE: Functional & Fit, Independent, Energized, Restored, Confident, Empowered

FIERCE: Functional & Fit, Independent, Energized, Restored, Confident, Empowered® promotes the benefits of physical activity and movement during and after cancer treatment.

FIERCE came about through a need in my community for an active cancer support group. There were plenty of talk-support groups for people with cancer, but few involved physical activity, except several yoga classes for breast cancer survivors.

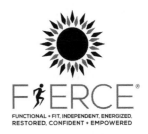

At a 5K race that raised funds for a non-profit called Hope Lives!, one of the runners told me she wished for just such a thing—a support group that included physical activity—and I decided to pursue it. Through the generosity of a local health club, Raintree Athletic Club, I started the FIERCE group in October 2014. It is free of charge to all cancer survivors in the community, and three years in, it is still growing.

I felt that cancer survivors in the community were missing out on the wonderful professional and skilled resources available in our town. There are a wealth of experienced and gifted coaches, instructors, and practitioners who were receiving few to no referrals from oncologists or physicians. The local cancer centers had resources for supervised rehabilitation services, but the FIERCE members were mostly beyond needing rehab. Many were done with treatment, or were going through it and desired to stay active and find support.

FIERCE meets twice a month in a beautiful, calming yoga studio. We begin with a warm-up of move-ment of major muscle groups, followed by stretching. I teach exercises that can be done without equip-ment, at home, with simple objects like a wall or a chair. Safety and balance are the priorities. Then we walk for 20 or 30 minutes.

The participants tend to pair off or form small groups according to their pace, which allows them to talk and support one another. The group is exceptional in varying their pace and the people they walk with, which creates an inclusive and welcoming environment for all. New participants are especially well-supported.

After that, we return to the athletic club and stretch more. For the second half of the class, we conduct either a question & answer session, wherein we all help each other find resources for our questions, or we listen to a demonstration by one of the many talented local practitioners. Demonstrations have come from yoga instructors, biofeedback practitioners, coaches and instructors in Pilates, Rossiter®, Feldenkrais®, Tai-Chi, Qi Gong, and other mind-body practices, as well as psychotherapists, counselors, registered dietitians, massage therapists, and more.

I personally meet with all presenters before I allow them to present to the class. I make sure they are knowledgeable and credentialed, professional, sensitive, and empathetic, as well as responsible in their promotion of their own modalities and any benefits they claim.

Introducing the FIERCE members to these healing modalities and experts in the community gives them a broader understanding of the importance of movement and its benefits, as well as the variety of ways to increase physical activity and enjoy movement. They also engage in healthy behaviors that may improve their quality of life and reduce their risk of cancer recurrence. It also supports the local community, which has a rich assortment of resources for cancer survivors that provide benefits beyond clinical and medical interventions.

For community providers who are interested in implementing FIERCE or want to learn more about the FIERCE curriculum, exercises, requirements, and structure, please visit the Cancer Harbors website contact page at https://cancerharbors.com/contact/.

Why the FIERCE acronym?

Functional & Fit	When people engage in physical activity and exercise, they are healthier and function better in their everyday lives.
Independent	People who have higher levels of fitness stay independent longer and are able to do more for themselves.
Energized	Physical activity gives energy, and fatigue is one of the most common effects of cancer treatment.
Restored	Physical activity returns people to normal lifestyle behaviors and social energy. Physical exercise also boosts cognitive health by regenerating new neural cells in the part of the brain that creates functional connections. A frequent unwanted effect of cancer treatment is "chemo brain." When physical activity is combined with cognitive training, these activities can improve people's cognitive function. Further, during exercise, the body produces hormones called endorphins. Endorphins make people feel better, minimize pain and fatigue, and put them in a better mood.
Confident	Physical activity is a great confidence builder! It makes people use their body and all its parts. For those who have had surgery or treatments that affect the way they use their body, being able to use those parts and gain strength and function builds their confidence. That shows on the outside.
Empowered	When people are physically fit, they function better, think more clearly, feel good about themselves, need less help, feel more in control of their life, and simply feel better. They call the shots again!

The benefits of exercise related to cancer[1]

Can you really afford not to exercise?

Reduces circulating hormones associated with cancer growth (insulin, estrogen)	Decreases inflammation
Improves blood pressure and circulation	Lowers blood sugar
Reduces stress, anxiety, and depression	Improves mood
Gives energy and reduces fatigue	Reduces constipation
Improves sleep quality	Builds bone strength
Helps control weight	Reduces muscle and joint aches via endorphins
Improves appetite and enjoyment of food	Improves body composition: decreases fat and increases lean muscle mass
Associated with reduced risk of many chronic diseases, such as cardiovascular disease and diabetes	

---

1   (Campbell, 2012)

Alene Nitzky

The Lemonade Routine

Exercises to do in bed

There is ample and growing scientific evidence that exercise is important during cancer treatment. The American College of Sports Medicine, the American Cancer Society, and the National Cancer Institute all suggest that even on your worst days, as little as 10 minutes of gentle activity is beneficial (Campbell, 2012).

I developed the following exercise routine for a patient who was at the end of her life, yet she wanted to exercise. She had always been active and continued to walk her dog up to the last few weeks of her life. She asked me what she could do on the days she was unable to get out of bed.

I called it the Lemonade Routine, as in making lemonade out of lemons… If you can get through this routine, even if you experience several bad days in a row, you will not lose as much fitness as you would by doing nothing.

By doing this routine, you will bring more blood flow and oxygen to your muscles, and may bring more oxygen to the tumor, possibly increasing the likelihood of killing cancer cells (McCullough, Stabley, Siemann, & Behnke, 2014). You will improve circulation and bowel function, reduce the risk of developing blood clots, increase range of motion, strengthen your appetite, lessen your fatigue, and best of all, congratulate yourself on accomplishing something, even when you could not get out of bed for normal activities.

The entire routine takes about twelve minutes. Repeat each exercise for a full minute. Two-sided exercises should be done for 30 seconds per side.

References

Campbell, K. L. (2012). Benefits of physical activity after a cancer diagnosis. In Irwin, M. L. (Ed.), *American College of Sports Medicine: ACSM's guide to exercise and cancer survivorship* (pp. 49-71). Champaign, IL: Human Kinetics.

McCullough, D. J., Stabley, J. N., Siemann, D. W., Behnke, B. J. (2014). Modulation of blood flow, hypoxia, and vascular function in orthotopic prostate tumors during exercise. *Journal of the National Cancer Institute, 106*(4). doi:10.1093/jnci/dju036

The Lemonade Routine
Exercises to do in bed

Watch the YouTube instructional video at https://www.youtube.com/watch?v=VCtD0RBRNWg

1	**Grips**	Holding a soft object in your hand, such as a washcloth, squeeze for 2-3 seconds, then relax. Repeat for 30 seconds, then switch sides.
2	**Reverse crunch**	Place your hands under your low back. Gently press down, tilting your pelvis forward. Lift both legs, bringing your knees toward your chest, then lower your feet back to the bed. Repeat for 1 minute.
3	**Heel/toe pointers**	Lying down with your legs extended, pull your toes toward your head, then push your toes away toward the foot of the bed. Repeat for one minute.
4	**Leg lifts**	Lying on your back, lift one leg off the bed at a time, then return to the starting position. Switch legs. Continue alternating between legs for a full minute.
5	**Side leg lifts**	Lying on your side, lift your upper leg off the bed as high as you can, then slowly return to the starting position. Repeat for 30 seconds, then switch sides.
6	**Snow angels**	Lying on your back, extend your arms and legs, bringing them away from your body and back toward the center like a snow angel. Repeat for one full minute.

The Lemonade Routine

Exercises to do in bed

7	**Arm cross**	Lying on your back, extend your arms to the sides. Raise your arms, keeping them straight, and cross them over your body, then return to the starting position. Repeat for a full minute.
8	**Push and press**	Lying on your back with your knees bent, place your hands at your sides. Press into the bed with your hands until you feel a contraction in your chest, shoulders, and triceps. Hold for several seconds, then relax. Repeat for a full minute.
9	**Single leg heel slides**	Lying on your back with your knees bent, extend one leg, sliding your heel along the bed, then return to the starting position. Switch sides. Continue alternating sides for one full minute.
10	**Butterflies**	Lying on your back with your knees bent and your knees and heels together, slowly lower your knees to the sides. Return to the starting position. Repeat for one full minute.
11	**Bridges**	Lying on your back with your knees bent and arms at your sides, lift your hips off the bed without arching your back, keeping the weight of your upper body on your shoulders. Hold at the top for 5-10 seconds each time, then lower your hips to the bed. Repeat for one full minute.
12	**Shrugs**	Sitting up in bed, shrug your shoulders backward slowly for 30 seconds. After 30 seconds, switch directions, shrugging your shoulders forward for 30 more seconds.

Cancer Harbors

The Cancer Harbors program serves as a guide and resource during the early transition from cancer patient to cancer survivor. It helps with recovery from the effects of treatment, as well as restoring quality of life.

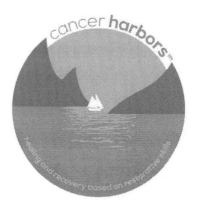

The program is intended to be started within six months of completing treatment for cancer, but can be used at any time after treatment. It is designed to last six months during the early recovery process, completing one section per month, with coaching and discussion around the topics of concern to the person using it.

The program contains six parts, listed on the next page. Sample modules from each part are included. Visit the Cancer Harbors website at cancerharbors.com for additional information.

Cancer Harbors sample modules	
Part 1	**Post-treatment**
	After cancer treatment: Important things to know
Part 2	**Physical activity, nutrition, and weight control**
	Healthy foods vs. healthy diet
Part 3	**Self-care and restoration**
	De-stressing from distressing
	A self-care exercise
Part 4	**Mental and emotional health and support**
	Emotional needs and support
Part 5	**Self-advocacy and health literacy**
	Taking responsibility for your health
Part 6	**Goals, personal growth, and moving forward**
	Goal-setting and reframing
Additional content available at cancerharbors.com	

Part 1: Post-treatment

Important things to know

Finishing chemotherapy, radiation, or surgeries, or whatever you consider to symbolize the end of cancer treatment, is not always a happy time. Ending treatment also opens the door to the unknown and to no longer being under the careful watch of your oncologist. Fear of being lost and feeling abandoned are common emotions during this time. Relieving that anxiety and regaining trust in your body takes time.

If you feel that your body betrayed you with cancer, it also takes time to relearn what various feelings and symptoms mean. Fear of recurrence might never go away, but you will become reacquainted with your body well enough so eventually you will not think every ache or pain is cancer.

Keep an open a line of communication with your oncologist on how you are feeling, but remember that your primary care physician can handle most issues. Stick to your follow-up appointments, scans, labs, and tests. They will make you anxious as they approach, but they are necessary.

Cancer Harbors is here to teach you skills to help you succeed at being as healthy, happy, and independent as possible as you move forward after treatment. Read through the sections, watch the videos, make a plan, talk to coaches, and get support in your community.

Use the checklists and hold yourself and your doctors accountable. Advocate for yourself. An active group with a concept like FIERCE can support you as you work through the early recovery period.

Recovering from cancer treatment and rebuilding trust in yourself can take months, or even years, as some of the treatment effects go away; others may never completely go away. The important thing is not to expect too much of yourself, especially in the first year or two after completing treatment.

It will take time for your body to recover from the drugs, treatments, and surgeries. Generally, the more treatments you had, the longer it takes to recover. It will take time for the lingering effects to fade, and then you will have a better idea of what still needs to be resolved. Everyone is different, so take what others tell you with a grain of salt. Some people recover more slowly or more completely than others.

If you were very active or athletic before your diagnosis, you might feel some frustration at the slow pace to regain fitness. If you were anemic during treatment, it takes time for your red blood cells to regenerate in adequate numbers so your body can deliver enough oxygen to your heart and muscles. If you lost muscle mass, it takes time to rebuild that, too.

Patience, especially with yourself, is the hardest part. It may seem unfair that you went through treatment and you're still not feeling as well as you want to.

Other people might try to dictate how fast you recover, but do not let them. No matter what your spouse, kids, friends, coworkers, or boss think, you are not just going to bounce back. Do not expect yourself to, and don't let them imply that you should be feeling better faster than you are. If you take on too much at first, you will set yourself back with fatigue, get sick from taxing your still-weak immune system, or possibly cause more cognitive difficulties while trying to recover function from chemo brain.

Remember, most people have no idea what it feels like to go through cancer treatment, so they will not understand what it is like afterward. Truly supportive people will listen to you, change their ways if you help them understand, and stick with you despite the rough times. Many people find that other cancer survivors become great friends because they can relate to what you have been though. It doesn't mean you have to talk about cancer all the time, or at all, but having that shared experience and mutual understanding can be an enormous source of comfort and support.

Expect to be supported, and do not allow people to treat you differently than you want to be treated. Don't allow people to dismiss where you are, even if you are afraid they will think you are using cancer as an excuse. You may not feel like the same person in some ways, and they should not expect you to be.

Healing takes place on many more levels than physical. Doing everything you can to take care of yourself from here on will ensure that you are living the best possible quality of life.

Part 2: Physical activity, nutrition, and weight control
Healthy foods vs. healthy diet

There is so much advice about eating, nutrition, supplements, and food, it can lead to confusion about what to do. It seems that every day there is a new product, superfood, or diet being advertised.

To reduce some of this confusion, ask yourself: What is a healthy food, and what is a healthy diet?

A single food might be considered healthy if it has qualities that are necessary for good health: high in vitamins and minerals and low in sugar, sodium, unhealthy fats, and calories. But this is only a small part of the picture. A food can contain important nutrients, but also unhealthy components. For example, a breakfast sandwich at a fast food restaurant might contain protein, carbohydrates, fat, and some vitamins and minerals, but it can also contain high amounts of sodium, saturated and trans fats, added sugar, and more calories than you need at the moment you eat it.

Kale, as another example, is considered a healthy food. It is high in calcium, B vitamins, vitamin K, and other vitamins and minerals. But if you ate only kale, you might end up with too much vitamin K (which can cause blood clotting), too much oxalate intake (which could lead to kidney stones), and too much fiber (which causes bloating and diarrhea).

Similarly, avocados are high in a number of vitamins, potassium, fiber, and healthy fat. If you were to eat nothing but avocados, however, you would be taking in all fat and no carbohydrates. Strawberries are low in sugar as far as fruits go, and they are high in vitamin C, but they contain no protein, no fat, and only a tiny amount of other nutrients.

A healthy food, by itself, is only healthy if it is part of an overall eating routine that contains many different healthy foods, each of which contributes to the nutritional quality of the whole diet. A healthy diet is not the same all the time. It provides the major nutrients your body needs (fat, carbohydrates, protein, fiber, vitamins, and minerals) in the right proportions, and it is not excessive or inadequate in amount or type of these nutrients.

Extreme diets or eating plans that are restrictive in which foods you can eat are not healthy diets. You should be free to eat any food. Portion sizes, caloric intake, and a variety of nutrients all contribute to a healthy diet.

Some of the popular "diets" contain healthy foods but restrict nutrient intake in certain areas. You do need some carbohydrates, preferably from whole grains, but eating too many grains can lead to nutrient deficiencies. Too many carbohydrates and not enough protein and fat can lead to hunger and weight gain. Too much protein is hard on the kidneys. Too much fat is hard to digest and can lead to weight gain. If your diet is restricted to too few foods, you will end up deficient in some nutrients and have an excess of others. That is not healthy.

Avoid the mindset that if something is good, then more is better. If something is good, include it along with other good things. You need balance in the types of foods you eat to cover the spectrum of necessary nutrients. It is better to eliminate the items that contain little nutritional value for the calories consumed: added sugar, trans fats, simple carbohydrates, processed and prepared foods, high sodium, and alcohol, all of which can lead to poor health when consumed too often or in great amounts. Choosemyplate.gov gives excellent visual images of healthy diets.

Don't restrict yourself from occasionally indulging in your favorite foods or beverages just because they are less healthy. What matters is how much and how often you consume them. If you eat good foods most of the time, you will not be harmed by indulging on occasion. It is easier to maintain a healthy diet without restrictions, which are mentally hard and can lead to cravings, binges, and other unhealthy eating behaviors.

If you would like additional help developing a healthy diet, find a local registered dietitian (R.D.) with at least Master's-level training, preferably with special training in oncology nutrition.

If your unhealthy eating habits might be behavioral in nature, consider seeking help from a counselor. If you ever feel out of control with your eating, contact a mental health practitioner who specializes in eating disorders. Your family doctor will be able to refer you.

How to take action

1   **Make a list of the foods you like that are healthy.** Buy these regularly when you are grocery shopping.

2   **Make a list of foods you should avoid (or have only occasionally).** Don't buy these at the grocery store (except on special occasions). When you go shopping for groceries, keep these lists with you—for example, on your phone.

3   **Take a special trip to the grocery store to look over the produce, fish, and meat sections, then the condiments, ethnic sections, and any other aisle that is not loaded with junk food.** Give yourself a chance to browse over the different items that are available. Don't get into a habit of always buying the same things and forgetting what other foods are available to you. Make a list of healthy items (from the entire store) that you would like to try in recipes.

4   **Make a list of all the fresh vegetables and fruits you haven't tried, and buy a new one each time you go to the store.** Go online and find recipes for these items. For example, if you want to try jicama (pronounced HE-ca-ma), search the term "easy jicama recipes" to give you ideas to start. Some websites, like epicurious.com or its app, are useful in this regard. Plan recipes around your healthy list. Make sure you choose foods from throughout the list of healthy foods.

5   **Do not keep unhealthy foods around the house.** If your weakness is ice cream, do not buy ice cream or keep it in the house. If you really want ice cream, make yourself go out and get it at an ice cream shop. You are buying only a portion for immediate consumption. (No leftovers!)

6   **If you are a meat eater, try planning your meals around vegetables.** Decide which vegetable you want as your main course, then choose the meat according to that. This forces you to think about the meal differently and can lead to healthier choices.

A word about sugar. Sugar, for reasons that are not entirely conclusive, may activate reward pathways in the brain in a similar manner to addictive drugs. This may be a survival mechanism, or there may be other explanations (Avena, Rada, & Hoebel, 2008; Brownell & Gold, 2012).

7   If you consider yourself to be addicted to sugar because you have it every day, start eliminating it from your diet and drinks. Avoid substitute sweeteners, too. It takes adjusting to the taste, but you can start to like foods without sugar. Then pay attention to your energy levels throughout the day compared to when you did eat sugar.

If you again try foods with added sugar after a few weeks without, you'll be surprised by how overly sweet things taste. You might prefer foods without sugar.

References

Avena, N. M., Rada, P., & Hoebel, B. G. (2008). Evidence for sugar addiction: Behavioral and neurochemical effects of intermittent, excessive sugar intake. *Neuroscience Biobehavioral Reviews, 32*(1): 20-39. doi:10.1016/j.neubiorev.2007.04.019

Brownell, K. D. & Gold, M. S. (2012). *Food and addiction: A comprehensive handbook.* New York: Oxford University Press.

Part 3: Self-care and restoration
De-stressing from distressing

Undergoing cancer treatment and the follow-up phase are stressful times. You might experience lack of coordination of your healthcare services, lack of communication between your healthcare providers, insurance coverage denials, financial concerns, or other aggravations that disrupt the process of getting to the services you need to feel better.

On top of that, a number of other concerns can add stress to the cancer experience: worrying about recurrence, worrying about the future and the unknown, difficulty accepting permanent changes to your body, and feeling like you don't have enough energy to do everything you need to.

In response to stress, the body releases chemicals that can affect your blood sugar or make your brain feel foggy, as well as other effects you don't want in a body healing from cancer.

The words *stress* and *management* are often found together, but not in a way that results in reduced stress. Management of anything can be stressful. Management implies you can control or influence the outcome of something, but not everything can be managed.

There has been much written about stress management, and most of it requires you to spend time, money, energy, or brain power to think about it or do it. What we really need is de-stressing from things that are distressing.

What can you do to de-stress?

1   **Ask for help.** Many people are too proud to admit they need help but find themselves needing help anyway. The act of asking for help then becomes another stressor. Remember, it is <u>not</u> a sign of weakness; in fact, it shows strength. A friend of mine who is a breast cancer survivor, athlete, and physician suggested there be a support group for those who are convinced they don't need support.

2   **Stop thinking.** When you find yourself feeling overwhelmed, catch yourself, stop your thoughts, and breathe slowly and deeply for several minutes, trying to clear your mind. The problems will be there after you take a break, and so will you.

3   **Practice letting go of worrying about the unknown.** There is nothing you can do to control it, beyond taking good care of yourself in the moment and being as consistent as possible. Don't expect perfection. You cannot control everything. It is stressful to try to control things you cannot control.

4   **Find new strengths in changes to your body.** Start by learning more about how your body works. As you find new ways to move, you will become aware of your muscles and new ways to strengthen your mind and body to support you in overcoming a loss of function. Physical and occupational therapists are invaluable in helping you discover how to compensate for movement restrictions.

5   **Find ways to decrease the burden on you.** These may be the burdens of work, things to do at home, and demands on your energy and time. Say no, and be assertive about what you need.

6   **Try yoga, mental imagery, deep breathing, relaxation techniques, biofeedback, massage, or exercise for 20-30 minutes a day.** These techniques can help you think more clearly, sleep better, and improve immune function. They require "me time." Do it regularly. Make it a habit. Assert yourself. You need it, and you deserve it.

7   **Keep a feeling-good file.** Include affirmations, such as thank you notes from others, statements of how you did a good job at something, or other things you are proud of. These are reminders of why you keep doing what you do. These are affirmations of self-worth and can help if you look over them on a bad day.

Refer to the Cancer Harbors modules on diaphragmatic breathing, exercise, and journaling and expressive therapies (https://cancerharbors.com/table-of-contents-cancer-harbors/) for more information on these suggestions.

Part 3: Self-care and restoration
A self-care exercise

Self-care is not about being selfish or self-absorbed. It is necessary for optimal health and well-being. It means you have a balanced, healthy relationship with people and things outside of yourself, as well as respect for yourself and your needs.

Self-care requires a healthy balance involving a certain amount of giving and taking. It means you exist in harmony with your inner and outer worlds, as a part of something bigger than yourself, while recognizing and accepting your own limits. The world places many demands on us, and when we add our own demands and expectations of ourselves, it's easy to be overwhelmed. We are so used to automatically multitasking through our days that most of us don't know what a healthy balance is.

What are the elements of our inner and outer worlds that need care? To simplify, think about these dimensions of your life: physical, social, emotional, spiritual, and mental, which includes occupation, intellect and learning, and creativity.

How do you take care of yourself in each of these areas, meeting your needs to the point where you are satisfied? Are there areas you have neglected or that need more attention than others?

To take care of yourself in each of these ways, think of the concepts of pampering, nurturing, and indulgence. You deserve to be treated with kindness, and sometimes you are the only one who will do so. As you think about these parts of your life, ask yourself how you can give yourself a gift in each of them.

Self-care ideas to consider

1   **Weed your garden.** If you have a caregiver type of personality (that is, you take care of others before yourself), assess how well those you are taking care of can do without you. If no harm will come to them without your involvement, it's a good sign you can let go. And for those people who truly suck the life out of you, it is time to "pull those weeds."

2   **Remember when you paid a price for overextending yourself.** Don't do it again.

3   **When others make demands on you, assertiveness is an asset.** *No* is not a four-letter word. Before adding anything else to your plate, take time to decide if it is a reasonable request and whether you truly want to do it. Listen to what you really want. Decline graciously the first time. After that, an emphatic "no" is warranted.

4   **"Me time" is not a luxury.** It's a necessity when you are recovering from an illness or stressful time. Who else can take care of your obligations, like watching the kids, while you nap?

5   **Experience healthy indulgences.** Go for a walk. Get exercise. Meet a friend who nurtures you for a cup of coffee or a glass of wine. Go to a museum, art gallery, or movie. At home, rearrange furniture or artwork in a room, or create something. If you can, go for a haircut, manicure, pedicure, massage, or spa visit. While exercise and diet are important priorities for your health, it's also okay to have a sugary or decadent treat every so often.

6 **Establish healthier relationships.** Recognize and stick with people who listen as well as talk, give as well as receive, don't demand anything of you when you're tired, and respect your schedule, needs, energy levels, and well-being. Discard those relationships that do the opposite—the sooner, the better.

7 **You don't need an excuse to focus on yourself.** Women, especially, neglect their own needs to focus on others. Take the time to reflect on what is important in life and what is not. You've just seen how life can change in the blink of an eye. Enjoy yourself and respect yourself. Listen to your needs, and don't let a chance to do that go by.

8 **Seek guidance from a mental health professional to help you with these suggestions and reframe your thoughts in a positive way if you are struggling.** Stress, depression, and anxiety make it difficult to see things in a positive light. There is nothing wrong with seeking help for your mental health; once you do, you might wonder why you waited so long!

Action: Self-inventory, present and future

A self-inventory is a helpful exercise every so often.

1. **List the elements of your world on the left side of the table. Add more dimensions of your life if you need to.**

	present needs	*future needs/consequences*
emotional		
spiritual		
physical		
social		
intellectual/ occupational/ creative		

2. **Do this exercise twice—once for how you feel about the present, and again while thinking about the future—at whatever time interval you choose.**

   Being in the present is very important, but you also must anticipate what your needs will be in the future, as well as the consequences of not facing the shortcomings in your life now.

3. **Use the suggestions throughout *Part 3: Self-care and restoration* to consider ways to improve your self-care.**

   This exercise can help you determine your priorities and the urgency of the need to make changes in self-care.

Part 4: Mental and emotional health and support
Emotional needs and support

Sadness, aloneness, anger, resentment, fear, and self-pity: These are real and very normal feelings about cancer. Allow yourself to feel and be with these emotions, as they will come and go. You need to give the feelings space to exist. If you can process them, you will move past them when something else distracts you.

You may experience feelings you don't feel comfortable expressing to those closest to you. Journaling and expressive therapies can be extremely helpful, as well as a support person or group to talk to.

When you have these feelings, it is important that they pass and do not interfere with your functioning. If you think they are interfering with your everyday tasks or relationships, seek help. Start with your doctor if you don't know who else to ask for help. Even though your doctor may not be able to address your specific mental health concerns, he or she can steer you in the right direction. Social workers, patient navigators, and counselors are available. Do not try to handle cancer alone.

Social support and communication are key. Many people have a hard time reaching out, and they struggle with the following issues:

» Gender expectations

» Communication skills

» Fear of showing vulnerability

» Not wanting to admit they don't understand something the doctor says

» A feeling of powerlessness

» Coping with traumatic events or intrusive thoughts

» Embarrassment and shame

Local support groups can be very helpful, especially at the beginning when you are in unfamiliar territory. As you begin to process your feelings, you may be able to manage them without being overwhelmed.

Support groups are most helpful when they focus on helping each individual move forward and cope with the multiple challenges that come with cancer. It is okay to vent and express your frustrations at times, but if your support group seems to only function as an outlet for venting and does not help you with your overall well-being and functioning, it is best to find another group that meets your needs.

Even if a local support group is not available to you, support groups of every stripe exist on social media platforms such as Facebook and Twitter, as well as elsewhere online, such as patient advocacy websites, nonprofit foundations' websites, discussion groups, and chat rooms.

The point is, you do not have to be alone in your feelings. Cancer can be very isolating, especially if no one in your immediate social circle has experienced it, or if you're in a rural area or small town with limited support resources.

While many medical websites or cancer center websites provide good information, they often skim over individual lifestyle needs and concerns. That's why patient advocacy organizations are so important: They help you connect with other patients and survivors who have been through it and can support you in your real-life needs that go beyond medical treatment.

Please refer to the short list below to explore help that exists online. These are just a few starting places; the possibilities are endless. You can enter search terms in a social media site or your browser's search engine. If you are not familiar with using social media platforms such as Twitter, refer to the Cancer Harbors module, "Using Social Media & Tweetchats for Information & Support" (found at https://cancerharbors.com/table-of-contents-cancer-harbors/).

Twitter: #patientadvocacy

Websites not specific to cancer but helpful resources:

http://patientadvocate.org

http://survivorshipatoz.org

http://themighty.com

Part 5: Self-advocacy and health literacy
Taking responsibility for your health

If you've gone through cancer treatment, you know that being a patient can be a full-time job. But you might also have learned that vigilance on your part can make all the difference.

Healthcare is too big and complex an industry now; you simply cannot take a passive role and let care be done to you. Too many important details slip through the cracks. Electronic health records do not guarantee that everything will be taken care of automatically. Even though this system is very different from 20 years ago, it is still run by, dependent upon, and in the service of humans.

Health literacy

We all need a certain amount of understanding of our bodies, diseases, and healthcare, and how they work and interact. Everyone will be a patient at some point in their lives. Most of us started life as a patient, and many of us will end it the same way.

You cannot control everything about your health, but you can control a lot. You can control how you take care of yourself and how you learn about your own health conditions and your family history. You can control how you interact with your doctors and other healthcare providers, by following their recommendations and communicating with them when something is not working.

Health literacy, in a practical sense, is knowing what you need to know about your health when you need to know it. It is also about how and where to learn what you need to know. There is an enormous amount of information on the Internet about health. At first, it's a good idea to avoid .com sites. They often contain conflicting and untested information. Major medical organizations with cancer centers, such as Dana Farber, M.D. Anderson, Mayo Clinic, and Fred Hutchinson, are usually better choices for information. After you understand how to recognize good information, you can explore .com sites, but continue to consume the information cautiously.

Martine Ehrenclou's book, *The Take-Charge Patient*, is also an excellent resource. I highly recommend this book to all because everyone will interact with the healthcare system eventually. For further learning, refer to the Prevent-Prepare-Prehab section (page A46) for more information on what you should know and do before you are ever diagnosed with a serious illness.

Confidence and assertiveness

It takes a certain amount of confidence and assertiveness to interact with doctors and the healthcare system because it moves quickly, communicates in big words and technical language, takes a lot of time, costs a lot of money, and can mean the difference between life and death. It can be intimidating, especially when you are scared and overwhelmed.

Even if you are already a naturally confident or assertive person, a physical examination can be intimidating. Being examined by a doctor, especially one you have never met before, can make you feel vulnerable or humiliated. You may be less likely to ask questions and assert yourself because all you want to do is get dressed and get out of there. Be aware that you might respond this way and remember you still must stand up for yourself.

Practice telling doctors when you are having a hard time. Do not minimize your symptoms. Too many people give a knee-jerk response when asked, "How's it going?" Without thinking, they respond, "Fine," or "I'm good," and the doctor quickly moves on to the next question. It's okay, and necessary, to be honest. Don't worry about making the doctor uncomfortable or staying a little longer. The only way you have a chance to get help is if you tell your doctor what is wrong.

During treatment, you had very little control, and treating cancer was a full-time job. After treatment, you can take a little more control; your life is no longer governed by juggling appointments. Assert your need to take care of yourself, including when you make your doctor appointments. Otherwise you will find yourself back in that place where you were controlled by cancer.

After you have been through cancer treatment, you may feel like more of an expert on healthcare. The anxiety you once felt about not knowing what was going to happen may be replaced by new feelings. There will still be anxiety about the unknown, but you will know what to expect during appointments. You will feel more confident about asking questions and knowing what you need to do to follow up.

Advocates

Bringing a health advocate along to appointments is a form of self-advocacy. The advocate should be assertive but let you speak and make sure your needs are addressed. Remember, it's about you, not the advocate.

Communication between doctors' offices and other providers

You need to make sure communication happens. When you are referred to a new doctor, make sure your records, labs, images, and other information arrive before your appointment. Check with the office staff in advance of your appointment, preferably by at least a day or two.

While most places now use electronic health records, many are incompatible with each other, especially when you move from one healthcare system or organization to another. That's another important reason to keep copies of records. Important information gets lost in the process of transferring from one place to another and ends up costing time, mostly yours. Know what information is being transmitted, to whom, and when.

You will have to do some checking on your own. Even with electronic communication, things slip through the cracks. You need a human to double-check. If you're waiting for a phone call from a doctor's office to schedule an appointment or give you your test results, find out when you should expect to hear from the office. If you don't get a call, follow up yourself.

Whenever your care must be coordinated among multiple doctors, directly ask your physician if he or she has spoken with the other doctors involved. This is very important for the quality of your care, for efficiency, and for setting expectations for the doctors. They will know you're on your toes, and they will know that you expect the same of them.

It's unfortunate that the healthcare system is fragmented in many ways, but to get the best care, sometimes you need to play the roles of detective and drill sergeant. Understanding the roles of various healthcare providers and staff can help you reach out for additional help when you need it. (Refer to page A39 for a description of their roles and how they can help you if you cannot get answers from a doctor.)

Before surgeries

Get specific information on your procedure so you can make informed decisions. Find out the success rate of your specific surgery by your surgeon, how many of the procedures he or she has done, how long the doctor has been in practice, and the infection rate of the facility, for this procedure and for surgeries performed by this doctor. Talk to other patients or people in the community to find out their impressions of the surgeon. Refer to Martine Ehrenclou's *The Take-Charge Patient* for further guidance on surgery.

Make sure hospital staff give you plenty of time and attention to discuss the surgery before you have it—not on the day of the surgery when you'll be tired, hungry, nervous, or groggy.

Ask:

» What can I do to ensure I have the best outcome?

» Is there anything I can do to prepare for the surgery (like prehab exercises)?

» How much pain can I expect to be in and for how long?

» Who can I call after hours if I have a question?

» How long will I be limited in my activities, or unable to work, and when can I expect to return to my normal activities?

Don't allow yourself to be rushed into decisions about surgery. Cancer is rarely an acutely life-threatening event. You will need time to gather yourself and your emotions and find support as you face major health decisions.

With plastic surgery, such as breast reconstruction, you do not have to do it right away or choose to do it at all. You might need time to think about how it will affect your long-term quality of life. The surgeon removing the cancer is not an expert in reconstruction. See a plastic surgeon to get the best advice on reconstruction. An excellent resource for breast reconstruction information is the Diep C Foundation at www.diepcfoundation.org.

Know your family history

This is some of the most important information you can provide to a doctor and can save you a lot of trouble. Hereditary mutations only account for a small percentage of cancers, but do bring it up if you have a family history of cancer.

This is also important for health concerns besides cancer, even for those not proven to be inherited mutations. I experienced this myself when trying to get a diagnosis for what turned out to be thyroid disease. I am the oldest of my generation in the family, and none of my parents or older relatives ever mentioned the fact they took thyroid medication. When I finally found out I had Hashimoto's thyroiditis, an autoimmune disease of the thyroid, the first thing my dad said was, "Oh, I've taken thyroid medication for years!" If I had known, it might have saved me a couple of years of banging my head into brick walls.

Respect your health and your body

You can guard your physical and psychological well-being by respecting your health and your body. You've been through too much already. Exercise, eat right, don't smoke, avoid too much alcohol, stay within your capabilities with your work and personal obligations, and don't take on more than you can handle. Stick to your follow-up checkups and scans. Take the medications your doctor prescribed because you agreed to take them.

Seek and accept psychological and emotional support

Some people feel they have to be strong all the time and are afraid if they let down their guard for a second, the cancer will come back. These people should give themselves permission to ask for help.

You simply cannot go through this entire process alone. Finding ways to support yourself is a part of self-advocacy.

During and after treatment, don't expect too much of yourself. Fatigue, chemo brain, and a weak immune system can last a long time.

You'll need to re-educate friends, loved ones, and coworkers; you might not feel like the same person, and they should not expect you to be. Many awkward moments can occur because of this misunderstanding. Remember, most people have no idea what it feels like to go through cancer treatment, so they will not understand what it is like afterwards.

If the things people say bother you, you can write about them in a journal or discuss them with someone you trust. That's a good way to vent. People will tell you you're strong and use other battle language. You may not be bothered by it, or you may dislike the clichéd association with a battle that is so common with cancer. Some people don't want to be strong all the time. Supportive people will allow you to have your moments when you don't feel like a fighter and don't want to be called one. You don't have to be a fighter. Refer to the Cancer Harbors module, "Dealing with Difficult People," found at https://cancerharbors.com/table-of-contents-cancer-harbors/, for more guidance.

It can be difficult to talk with people who can't seem to get past the topic of cancer when they see you, but try not to isolate yourself. It's okay to feel like you don't want to see anyone, but isolating yourself can make life seem gloomy. There are certain people you might not want to be around, but allow others to visit. People will want to support you, and you can decide whether to give them the opportunity.

Medications

If you have questions about medications, a pharmacist is a great resource. They are very knowledgeable about drugs and can provide information on side effects, interactions with other medications, and safety profiles. Pharmacists can also give you tips on how to keep track of your medications.

When you pick up your prescription medication, make sure the correct name (some are spelled or sound alike), dosage, instructions, and prescribing physician are on the label.

Make sure you understand the instructions before you leave the doctor's office or pharmacy. Do I need to take it with food? How many times a day do I need to take it? Should I take it before bed? Will it make me drowsy, or more alert? Could it interact with anything else I'm taking? Is it the same as anything else I'm taking? How long do I need to keep taking it? Do I need to finish the entire container? Do I need to stop this medication before any tests, surgeries, or procedures?

The following points on medication are important to your health and are your responsibility.

» Inform your doctor about everything you take, including supplements, over-the-counter medications, vitamins, herbs, and anything else you put in your body.

» Make sure the pharmacy knows your drug allergies.

» Make sure every doctor you see knows every medication every other doctor has prescribed. Discuss them even if they are already in your medical record. Many drugs have interactions. For example, Tamoxifen®, a drug used in treating breast cancer, interacts with certain antidepressants, and blood thinners. Certain supplements or herbs can interact with each other.

» When you travel, bring an extra supply of your medications in case you have a change in your travel plans. Always refill prescriptions ahead of time.

» Don't stop taking any medication without first discussing it with your doctor.

Don't 'wait 'til Monday'

If you are having symptoms or trouble, even if you are unsure whether they are related to treatment, let your doctor know. Many people are afraid to bug the doctor, or don't want to be seen as a wimp, complainer, or hypochondriac, but doctors need to know how you are responding to the treatment. If a drug is becoming too toxic, you might need a dose change or even a different medication. This is why there are on-call and after-hours numbers. Don't suffer, and don't wait until Monday to call the doctor.

Discussing death and advance directives

The topic of death is uncomfortable for most people, including doctors. It is a fact of life for everyone, however. If you have not discussed it with your family and doctors, do it.

It is okay to ask your doctor, "How long can I expect to live?" For some people, this is important in guiding their decisions and their outlook on life, while others may not care to go anywhere near that question. But remember, doctors can only estimate based on data and statistics. Everyone's outcome is different. Your doctor can't see into the future any better than you can.

Everyone should have advance directive legal documents[1] in place regardless of cancer status. They will describe your wishes in the event of severe illness or injury, when you cannot speak for yourself. Advance directives state who you want to make decisions for you when you are unable, and what you want for treatment or attempts to prolong your life. Setting up these documents is not a sign of giving up

---

1   The AARP provides information and explanations to start from: https://www.aarp.org/caregiving/financial-legal/info-2017/living-will-power-of-attorney.html

hope; instead, it's a gift to the people closest to you. It can be liberating to know that your needs will be taken care of no matter what happens.

Give these advance directives to your doctors, make sure your medical power of attorney knows what you want and has copies, and make sure these documents can be retrieved promptly when needed.

Death is a fact and a reality, something that will eventually happen even if you never have a cancer cell. Considering death can help you appreciate life and think about how you want to live the days you have. It can guide the decisions you make about your treatment, maintenance therapies, and how you want to take care of yourself for the rest of your life.

Roles of medical staff and healthcare personnel

Nurses and physicians are supported by numerous other staff. The roles of other medical staff that cancer patients may encounter are described below.

Medical assistants are trained in administrative and clinical tasks, such as record-keeping, taking medical histories, and vital signs. They may assist the doctor or nurse with certain procedures, but generally, they are not trained in the disease process or pharmacology and as such do not administer medications, interpret test results, or give medical advice. They report to an office manager or a licensed healthcare professional.

Nurse navigators are usually nurses or social workers who address a variety of patient needs, such as referrals to resources in healthcare facilities or the community that can make the patient's experience less stressful and more successful. They coordinate care, appointments, and communication among doctors, educate patients, and find financial assistance.

Forward-thinking healthcare facilities have begun to incorporate nurse navigation services automatically when a patient is diagnosed with cancer. The earlier the patient is connected to these services, the more advantageous they are for minimizing the patient's stress around the cancer treatment experience.

Dietitians are another beneficial healthcare provider for cancer patients. Many patients struggle to consume adequate calories when food is unappealing due to nausea. Doctors are not trained in nutrition and do not have time to discuss it at length, but they can refer patients to registered dietitians, who can help patients improve their nutritional intake.

Social workers coordinate the psychological and social needs of patients. They are often trained as mental health professionals or counselors, and they also have access to community resources, like navigators do. Social workers sometimes help patients find legal assistance, financial aid, child care, rides, meals, and other resources in the community, and they provide support through counseling.

Case managers can be nurses or other healthcare professionals who connect patients and their families with resources to meet treatment goals. They help the patient and family locate and access these services and evaluate whether those services are meeting the goals of the treatment plan.

Pharmacists are an excellent resource for patients regarding medications. You can discuss medication questions with a pharmacist if your doctor, physician assistant, nurse practitioner, or registered nurse is unavailable. Be sure you are speaking to a registered pharmacist, though (not a pharmacy tech).

Part 6: Goals and moving forward
Goal-setting and reframing

Cancer treatment can change you physically and mentally. It can be difficult to cope with the loss of goals and activities that were important to you pre-diagnosis. They often seem unattainable after cancer. When something you were able to do easily before cancer is no longer easy or even possible, you may feel a sense of loss.

The following are several examples of these types of losses:

» An athlete who relied on upper body strength, but breast surgeries have resulted in being unable to train at the same level as before

» A career-oriented individual whose professional goals are challenged by chemo brain

» A woman whose fertility is lost, along with her dream of having her own children; meanwhile, her fear of recurrence hinders pursuing other ways of raising children

For highly goal-oriented people, it can be hard to find motivation without a goal. A problem with goals, however, is that they are not always appropriate for what we can reasonably accomplish. No matter your health status, if you set a goal that is too difficult, it will lead to feeling inadequate or that you will never be successful. Researchers have found that mindfulness approaches to setting new goals, and stopping the process of obsessing about old expectations, can be helpful for cancer patients (Schroevers, Kraaij, & Garnefski, 2008).

The feelings are important, not the goal

A certain amount of grieving your losses must be done, but you must identify the point at which you are stuck in negative feelings. Obsessing over something you can't have is not a productive use of your time or emotional energy.

At some point, you must refocus your energy on finding a way forward. Come back to the present and think about what you can do. Make a list of things that will help you switch into positive gear when you find yourself ruminating on what you have lost. With practice and awareness, you can train yourself to recognize negative feelings when they arise and use them to switch gears in a positive direction.

Building confidence

Confidence in your ability to accomplish a task or goal is known as self-efficacy. When you believe you will succeed, you are more likely to succeed.

To rebuild your confidence, break goals into many small steps. Each step should contain tasks that must be completed before moving on to the next step. You can build self-efficacy by working step-by-step to achieve a larger goal, without taking on too much at once. You should enjoy the task and feel comfortable doing it before proceeding. If you need help, work with others who have experienced similar feelings while learning how to proceed, and who will help you without judgment or awkwardness.

Moving forward and setting new, realistic goals

1 **First, acknowledge the loss and your feelings around that loss.** When you find yourself feeling sorry for yourself, allow yourself time to be with the feelings. Don't forget those feelings, as they will be an important part of moving forward.

2 **Identify the positive feelings you want to experience while pursuing a goal.** What feelings did you have while pursuing a past goal that made it so important to you?

3 **Identify activities you can do that will bring that feeling or another equally positive feeling.** What activities do you enjoy that you <u>can</u> do? What is it about those activities that causes the pleasant feelings?

4 **Make a list of tasks and activities you can focus on that will lead to pleasant feelings.** When you catch yourself ruminating, switch to one of the tasks on the list.

5 **As you come up with ideas for goals around those new activities, write them down.** You will soon have a new set of goals to work toward.

If you're struggling with reassessing your goals, ask a coach, counselor, therapist, or a non-judgmental friend (who will not impose his or her beliefs) for help.

References

Schroevers, M., Kraaij, V., & Garnefski, N. (2008). How do cancer patients manage unattainable personal goals and regulate their emotions? *British Journal of Health Psychology, 13(*3), 551-62. doi:10.1348/135910707X241497

Additional content at Cancerharbors.com

The entire contents of Cancer Harbors are too extensive to be included in this book. The remaining modules can be accessed separately, with or without guided coaching, by visiting the Cancer Harbors website at https://cancerharbors.com/table-of-contents-cancer-harbors/. Guided coaching is highly recommended to tailor the program to your individual needs, maximize your benefits, and save you time.

You do not have to be a cancer survivor to benefit from Cancer Harbors. Many of the modules contain information and skill-building that will help anyone take better care of their health and improve quality of life. The modules in the FIERCE and Prevent-Prepare-Prehab sections of the book are also included in the Cancer Harbors website content. The modules are updated frequently as scientific evidence-based recommendations change. A list of recommended readings can also be found on the Cancer Harbors website at https://cancerharbors.com/recommended-reading/.

Remaining Cancer Harbors modules available at the Cancer Harbors website

During treatment

Newly diagnosed with cancer: Important things to know

During cancer treatment: Important things to know

Anemia

Electrolytes

Nadir

Neutropenia

Thrombocytopenia

Understanding labs

Your veins and chemo

Post-treatment

Aromatase inhibitors: Holding yourself and your doctor accountable with a checklist

Home and everyday safety

Radiation therapy: Healing and aftereffects

Sleep

What to do about chemo brain and cognitive dysfunction

Symptoms

Joint aches

Neuropathy

Pain

Nutrition

Balancing energy

Caloric intake, food choices, and eating at home: Actions to take/checklist

Healthy foods vs. healthy diet

Supplements, diets, and fads

Weight loss, abdominal fat, emotions, stress, and sleep

Exercise and exercise routines

Exercise during chemotherapy and radiation: Precautions during active cancer treatment

Beginning weight-bearing for osteoporosis

Chair core routine

Exercise and physical activity: Understanding the difference

Exercises after breast surgery, with and without reconstruction

Full body warm-up routine

Understanding the language of exercise

Upper body warm-up routine

Function and health

Appearance and coping with functional changes

Diaphragmatic breathing

Lymphedema

Osteoporosis

Oral health and dental concerns with cancer

Understanding chemo brain and cognitive dysfunction

Mental health, emotional support, and self-care

A self-care exercise

Control

Coping with fatigue

What to do about anxiety

Dealing with difficult people

Facing fears and anxiety

Indoor restorative environments

Journaling and expressive therapies

Lifelong learning

Mental health and cancer: Depression, anxiety, and other conditions

Outdoor restorative environments

Time and energy conservation

Trauma, PTSD, and coping

Self-advocacy

Interpreting research studies reported in the media

Online and printed information for health consumers

Prevention, risk & cause

Self-advocacy, health literacy, learning, and personal growth

Self-advocacy in communicating with doctors about symptoms, side effects, and pain

Taking responsibility for your ongoing health

Using social media & Tweetchats

Workplace, occupational, financial, and legal considerations

Breast cancer-specific

Breast reconstruction options and resources

Living with aromatase inhibitors and Tamoxifen®

Managing side effects of aromatase inhibitors

Other cancer-related information

Fertility resources

Genetic counseling and testing resources

Sexuality resources

Prevent-Prepare-Prehab
Educating the Public

This section of the appendix is primarily aimed at those who have never had cancer. The Prevent-Prepare-Prehab program provides specific information to boost cancer literacy and build skills for interacting with the healthcare system. An educated public will be well-equipped to think clearly and calmly, find resources, and make informed decisions about healthcare when presented with a potentially life-threatening disease diagnosis.

Education, not just awareness

I am proposing this template as a preliminary model for educating the public in three areas: 1) preparing for interactions with the healthcare system, 2) minimizing trauma and shock in the event of a cancer diagnosis, and 3) increasing health and consumer literacy around cancer-related health products, services, and information. It is my hope that this curriculum will be introduced via public health efforts in conjunction with progressive healthcare reform. I propose knowing this information as a requirement for accessing universal healthcare, but there are many other ways it could be implemented.

Our current methods of mass education through cancer awareness campaigns, consisting of bright colors, short sound bites, and pink feathers and pom-poms, are inadequate or even misleading when it comes to building cancer literacy. These campaigns are often focused on making money and marketing products instead of building literacy and practical skills in prevention, preparation, and self-advocacy.

What we need instead is a focused, universal health curriculum about cancer that reaches everyone. Healthcare professionals cannot simply tell their patients to change their ways and expect success if they are not given the guidance, skills, and coaching to succeed. That's why this type of program is needed.

I have included some of the Prevent-Prepare-Prehab curriculum in this book, but it is far from complete. I offer this as a general place to begin. Throughout the text, I refer to numerous Cancer Harbors modules, which can be found at https://cancerharbors.com/table-of-contents-cancer-harbors/.

Alene Nitzky

The P-P-P curriculum

Prevent

I am frequently asked, "What is the single most important thing I can do to prevent myself from getting cancer?" While there is no absolute right answer that universally applies to everyone, there are certain behaviors that will protect you from chronic disease. While nothing you do is an absolute guarantee that you won't get cancer or a chronic disease, by following these guidelines, you will be more likely to live a longer and healthier life.

1   **Move**. Get plenty of regular physical activity, much more than the minimum recommended amount of exercise. The minimum amounts recommended for prevention (generally 150 minutes a week of moderately intense activity), in my opinion, are not enough! You need vigorous and sustained activity on a regular basis. Humans were made to move. Thirty minutes out of a 24-hour day (about two percent of the time!) won't put a dent in your health if you want to develop a level of fitness that will protect you from adverse health consequences. (See the Cancer Harbors and FIERCE modules for more information.)

2   **Eat in moderation, and nearly always high-quality food**. High-quality food contains the nutrients your body requires to fuel itself for everyday activities, as well as to repair and heal tissues. A variety of nutrients are required to fuel all of your body's processes: some tissues, such as your brain, need glucose (sugar), while your muscles, including your heart, need certain minerals to contract properly. Protein and fats are needed to repair tissues and produce hormones, among other vital processes. When recovering from an injury to the body, such as surgery, chemotherapy, or radiation, your body relies on high-quality foods to fuel the repair process. Your body cannot heal or recover as quickly when you are undernourished.

3 **Take care of your mental and emotional health needs.** Don't neglect your mental well-being; reach out for help <u>before</u> the stress of an illness makes mental health issues worse. Take care of those areas of your life that contribute to stress. (Refer to the Cancer Harbors module titled "De-stressing from Distressing" on page A24 for more information.)

4 **Take care of your personal safety.** Refer to the "Home and Everyday Safety" module at https://cancerharbors.com/table-of-contents-cancer-harbors/ for ideas on protecting yourself at home.

5 **Stay on top of your screenings for early detection (for example, colonoscopies).** Don't delay a trip to the doctor if you suspect something is wrong. Remember, screenings do not <u>prevent</u> cancer, but they do detect it early—often before intensive cancer treatment is needed. Screenings may also provide peace of mind when completed.

Prepare

No one is ever going to be prepared for hearing that they have cancer; there is an element of shock that accompanies this news from your doctor. There are many details you can prepare ahead of time, however, so you won't have to worry about them at a stress-filled and over-whelming time. Why not plan ahead to take the burden off you, your caregiver, and loved ones?

1   **Complete the Values Exercise** (page A8). This will help you set your priorities and align your behaviors with what is most important to you.

2   **Practice communicating with your doctors, nurses, and other healthcare provid-ers, every time you go for a medical appointment.** Try being more assertive about your needs. Ask questions. Even one question is better than keeping quiet. The Cancer Harbors module called "Communicating with Healthcare Providers" (page A59) will help you learn what questions to ask.

3   **Complete your advance directives and make sure they are in your medical records.** This a great way to practice being assertive with your doctor, which can lead to deeper conversations and establishing a better, more trusting relationship. Start by learning the basics at the AARP website: https://www.aarp.org/caregiving/financial-le-gal/info-2017/living-will-power-of-attorney.html.

4   **Find and designate an advocate and caregiver who will attend doctor appoint-ments with you, take notes, ask questions, and lend an extra pair of ears to listen.** The advocate and caregiver don't necessarily need to be the same person, but if they are not, they should both have good communication skills and a trusting working relationship, with your best interests foremost in mind. You, in turn, can offer to do the same for them, should they need it.

Learn more about health, and improve your health literacy and your reading comprehension of health journalism. As you become a more critical consumer of health products, services, and information, you will find it easier to discern good information from bad. Two places to start building these skills are:

» Health News Review (http://healthnewsreview.org)

» Center for Science in the Public Interest (https://cspinet.org/)

5 Guides are available to help you evaluate information you find online:

» MedlinePlus Guide to Healthy Web Surfing (http://www.nlm.nih.gov/medlineplus/healthywebsurfing.html)

» Evaluating Internet Health Information: A Tutorial from the National Library of Medicine (http://www.nlm.nih.gov/medlineplus/webeval/webeval.html)

» Health Insight (http://www.health-insight.com/; a humorous but informative site)

Read the Cancer Harbors module on taking responsibility for your health. This will help you know what questions to ask in case of a serious diagnosis. Prepare a

6 folder or binder to keep all your personal medical records and information in one place. Prepare a partial list of questions and keep it with your health information so it is easy to find when you need it.

Understand your insurance coverage. Keep insurance information with your medical

7 records. At the least, know where to find that information.

Keep track of all your surgeries, illnesses, hospitalizations, medical history, doctors, specialists, therapists, and other professional health contacts. Don't rely on doctors to do this for you. Medical records are full of inaccuracies. Make a date

8 with yourself every so often to update it—maybe yearly, or any time you have a new prescription, diagnosis, procedure, labs, or surgery. Then, make a habit of taking this information with you when you travel, and make sure your emergency contact person also knows where this information is.

9 **Make a list of all your medications, their purpose, how you take them (by mouth, patch on your skin, etc.), doses, frequency, and any allergies to medications.** If you can't find all this information, get it from your doctor or pharmacist. You can call to find out at any time. Keep this with your other medical information, and always take it with you to doctor appointments. Update it frequently.

10 **Think about the things you might want to change in your home, in case you or a family member were to become disabled, or what you'll want when you get older.** Imagine if you were in a wheelchair temporarily. Where in your home would you be able to go? What would you have trouble reaching? Imagine if you couldn't lift your arm over your head, stand, walk up and down the stairs, or lift an object heavier than a pound.

You can start rearranging things in your home so they are more accessible, to whatever extent you are able to do or afford. A good place to start is by visiting the website of The National Aging in Place Council at http://ageinplace.org.

11 **Learn, vote, and speak your mind.** Civic engagement is necessary to being an active, informed citizen. It is also a great way to give back to your community. Which health-related issues are most important to you? Take five to ten minutes each week to make a call or write a quick letter to your representatives or senators to let them know how you feel about a specific issue and how you would like them to vote. Volunteer at a public health agency if you have the time. A good place to start is the League of Women Voters, a non-partisan organization for both men and women: http://lwv.org/.

Prehab

You might be familiar with the term "prehab" if you have been around orthopedic surgeons or physical therapists. Short for prehabilitation, it is a program of exercises or educational material used before medical treatment to improve outcomes for patients after treatment, and to reduce health care costs and complications (American Academy of Orthopedic Surgeons, 2014; Corder, Kenner, Sherwood, Kusmierczyk, & Duval, 2015).

Prehab is simply doing whatever possible to prepare people before they go through treatment for their disease. It maximizes the likelihood that they will come through treatment better than if they had not prepared beforehand. Preparation can include many aspects of their lives: physical, mental, emotional, functional, and more.

Education is prehab, as is thinking ahead. The following guidelines, which are often given for general health and prevention, are considered prehab:

If you smoke, stop.
If you're overweight, lose weight.
If you eat a poor diet, improve your diet.
If you're sedentary, start exercising.

Prehab is a concept that is fairly new to oncology, but it has been demonstrated to be effective for lung cancer patients prior to surgery (Silver & Baima, 2013) and is being explored for other types of cancer treatments.

While prehab is not universally covered by insurance companies (American Physical Therapy Association, 2015), or even prescribed by doctors, you can do some prehab on your own. To prepare for a surgery or any other treatment, start by establishing clear communication with surgeons, doctors, nurses, physical or occupational therapists, and other professionals on your treatment team.

For many surgeries—breast reconstruction or hysterectomy, for example—prehab is certainly an important consideration. What does your body need to be prepared for surgery? Do you need to strengthen certain muscles? Do you need to make certain items in your home easier to reach so you will be more independent during recovery?

You can address emotional prehab on your own by asking yourself some questions: Do you have emotional support among people closest to you? Do they understand the process of treatment and the changes to your body, and how they will affect you emotionally and physically? Are they willing to be patient and accepting? Will they give you the time and space you need to cope with your treatment?

Why is prehab important?

Cancer is still so feared that we don't teach about what treatment requires of us. But you can prepare for faster recovery, with fewer complications, in part by being as healthy and active as possible all the time.

Upon the shock of a cancer diagnosis, some people rush into surgery, even when it may not be the best choice for them in the long run. But when you take time to think about your options and educate yourself, you will rely less on doctors to make decisions that will affect you for the rest of your life.

References

American Academy of Orthopaedic Surgeons. (2014, October 7). Can physical therapy before hip, knee replacement surgery improve outcomes? *Science Daily.* Retrieved February 17, 2016, from: www.sciencedaily.com/releases/2014/10/141007111225.htm

American Physical Therapy Association. (2015, August 5). Washington Post: 'Growing interest' in prehab for individuals with cancer doesn't translate into insurance coverage. *PT in Motion News.* Retrieved February 17, 2016, from: http://www.apta.org/PTinMotion/News/2015/8/5/PreHabWaPost/

Corder, M., Kenner, R., Sherwood, J. T., Kusmierczyk, C., Duval, K. (2015). Prehabilitation demonstrates decreased hospital length of stay in a small sample of thoracic oncology patients. In *Oncology Nursing Society Annual Congress: Podium and Poster Session Abstracts* (pp. 238-239). Pittsburgh, PA: Oncology Nursing Society. doi: 10.1188/15.ONF.E110

Silver, J. K., & Baima, J. (2013). Cancer prehabilitation: an opportunity to decrease treatment-related morbidity, increase cancer treatment options and improve physical and psychological health outcomes. *American Journal of Physical Medicine & Rehabilitation, 92*(8): 715-727.

Get started on Prevent-Prepare-Prehab now

What are you waiting for?

1   **Complete the Values Exercise.** (page A8)

2   **Read and learn.**

     » Taking responsibility for your health (page A32)

     » Cancer: Frequently asked questions (page A55)

     » Communicating with healthcare providers (page A59)

     » Prehab module (page A52)

3   **Get up and move.**
Make the changes you've been wanting to. Don't wait for a New Year to resolve to focus on health. Cancer Harbors can help you even if you don't have cancer.

4   **Make an action plan for completing the tasks in the Prepare section.**

5   **Contact Cancer Harbors for coaching guidance to get the most out of this information and start building healthy skills now.**

Cancer: Frequently asked questions

What is cancer, in a nutshell?

Cancer as we think of it is a complex and varied group of diseases, but the word *cancer* is a term for uncontrolled growth of cells that invade healthy tissue. There are hundreds of types of cancer, and each one behaves and responds differently within the body in which it grows. How we currently classify, stage, and treat cancer is based on our current understanding of what triggers or stops cancer growth. The most common treatments for cancer are surgery, chemotherapy, radiation, and newer treatments such as targeted therapies (also called biotherapies). Less commonly, bone marrow (stem cell) transplants are used to treat cancer.

The severity of a person's cancer is often described in stages, from 0 through IV, depending on to what extent the cancerous cells have invaded the tissue and spread to the lymph nodes or other parts of the body. Some cancers are not staged, or may have their own staging scheme.

What are some assumptions about cancer?

When I speak to groups, one assumption always arises: Each time, someone tells me they think they will never get cancer because they eat well, exercise, and do all the right things. To people who have had cancer, it sounds like they're being told they got cancer because they didn't take care of themselves.

Healthy privilege is a term that describes this assumption. When you are blessed with good health and have never faced a serious illness, it is easy to assume that the way you live is the right way. Since it works for you, you assume it should work for others. It's a nice, comfortable place to be. Those assumptions can get you in trouble, however.

The fact is, you do not know how you will feel or act until you are in the situation yourself. It is not fair to the person who is going through cancer to judge his or her choices or decisions. Instead, allow people to come to informed decisions on their own, with professional guidance, and then support them as they move forward.

My hope is that through Cancer Harbors, this book, and the resources here, we can cultivate a more productive level of health, cancer, and consumer literacy, and minimize the confusion that impairs our ability to make good decisions when we are faced with cancer.

What is alternative medicine for cancer?

Technically, "alternative" means you are using a treatment outside of standard medical therapies. If that alternative treatment happens to boast unproven claims of effectiveness, lacking randomized trials and a body of evidence to support its effectiveness, you are taking a big chance. One study is not a body of evidence, and it is not conclusive.

People often confuse complementary therapies with alternative medicine. Complementary therapies, such as massage and acupuncture, work in conjunction with standard medical cancer treatments like chemotherapy and radiation. Integrative medicine is a new field that researches these therapies. There is growing evidence that some are effective. Exercise, which I like to think of as a complementary therapy, has a substantial body of evidence for its effectiveness in improving function and quality of life (Schmitz et al., 2010).

Many chemotherapy drugs have been used for years on large numbers of patients and have been tested through randomized trials. We have a very good idea of how they work, what they can and cannot do, and what problems they cause in the short- and long-term. This is not to say that chemo and Western medicine are always effective, despite bodies of evidence to support their use.

If your doctor informs you that you need chemotherapy, it's not an ideal choice to face. But remember that it's your life, and your family, kids, parents, pets, or whomever love and depend on you. There is risk with any drug, Western or alternative, but wouldn't you choose the one that has been tested on much greater numbers of people?

Here is food for thought if you are ever diagnosed: "I don't like to take drugs" is not a good reason to delay treatment, because if you wait and your cancer becomes advanced, you may experience more pain, lose function, and have fewer options and less hope. You may lose the option to take drugs or recover from the cancer. I have seen many people delay conventional treatment in hopes that an alternative method will work, but end up back in the traditional healthcare system with advanced cancer that cannot be stopped.

For some people, no amount of information or evidence will change their minds if they are convinced they don't want to do something. This is one area where you don't want to make decisions beforehand, however, because every individual's cancer situation is different. If you have carefully weighed the risks and benefits and have adequate information about every option, you have every right to make an informed choice for yourself.

How can cannabis help cancer patients?

There are many (at least anecdotal) benefits of cannabis for pain, nausea, appetite, anxiety, and more. Given the issues with opioid use that have surfaced over the past several years, it appears that cannabis may be a promising alternative for relieving certain symptoms.

It is not a substitute for any chemotherapy drug, however, and if you are considering the use of cannabis while receiving chemotherapy or other forms of cancer treatment, ask your oncologist if it could harm you or reduce the effectiveness of the chemotherapy. When you are on chemotherapy or any mixture of drugs, it's like stirring a giant, steaming cauldron. Unless you know how what you're adding to the mix will react, you risk an explosion. Ask the chemist (your oncologist).

I hope cannabis will be the focus of more research in the coming years, and that physicians may become more comfortable with cannabis for symptom relief. For now, the tangle of legal issues and jurisdictions complicates cannabis research.

How do I talk to someone with cancer?

People feel uncomfortable with topics they fear or don't understand, especially around matters of life and death. Many people are afraid of their own mortality and have a difficult time being around those with cancer, even if the cancer is likely to be cured. But talking with people with cancer is a great way to gain understanding and empathy and overcome your fear.

You can simply listen, or ask what you can do for them right now. They probably do need something, and you would be there at just the right time to help. And if they don't need help, they will tell you. The Cancer Harbors website contains a guide (found at https://cancerharbors.com/anatomy/) for people who are uncomfortable in this situation.

What is Stage IV cancer, and does it mean the person will die?

The Stage IV designation means that the cancer has spread to areas of the body that are far from the original site. Generally, it can't be cured, but Stage IV cancer patients can have widely varying lengths of survival. It is possible to undergo treatment for years, or be in and out of treatment, to keep the disease under control. Do not assume people with Stage IV cancer are going straight into hospice care or will be saying their goodbyes soon. Not everyone with Stage IV cancer is imminently dying, and every individual is different in this regard. People with Stage IV cancer will, most likely, eventually die of the disease, rather than something else, but sometimes they live for many years and can achieve good quality of life during that time.

If you know people with Stage IV cancer, reach out to them; they will appreciate it. They might not want to talk about their illness, but people do cope and adjust over time. Express that you understand if they don't feel like talking, but that you would love to see them when they feel like it. They are still the same person, and your relationship doesn't need to stop because of their Stage IV cancer.

References

Schmitz, K. H., Courneya, K. S., Matthews, C., Demark-Wahnefried, W., Galvao, D. A., Pinto, B. M., et al. (2010). American College of Sports Medicine roundtable on exercise guidelines for cancer survivors. *Medicine and Science in Sports and Exercise, 42*(7), 1409-1426. doi:10.1249/MSS.0b013e3181e0c112

Alene Nitzky

Communicating with healthcare providers

Your relationship with and your trust in your doctor and their staff has a great impact on your outcome. Cancer is stressful enough; you do not need to add stress by having an uncomfortable experience every time you see the doctor. Understanding your doctor's scope of practice and how to best communicate with him or her can pave the way for smooth interactions whenever you receive care.

Expectations versus reality in healthcare

Don't expect everything of your doctor. Doctors are human, and there is only so much they can do in a day to give the care that each patient deserves. They have good days and bad days, as do their office staff, but if they act in your best interest and you feel safe, comfortable, and trusting in their care, you've probably found a good fit. You should never feel that you are just a number or labeled as a disease rather than the individual person you are.

Understand healthcare providers' scope of practice

Healthcare providers have different titles, roles, and something called scope of practice, which is what they are trained, educated, and licensed to do and practice under the law. Doctors are trained in medicine, which means diagnosing, treating, and prescribing medicine or medical interventions to treat or cure an illness.

Doctors practice medicine, nurses practice nursing care, ultrasound techs operate ultrasound machines, and housekeepers clean and sanitize patient rooms. A doctor who is asked to sanitize a patient room might not know the proper technique and would need to rely on the housekeeper for guidance. Scope of practice is often interpreted broadly for physicians, giving them a wide margin of freedom to recommend certain practices, but they are not experts on all topics they may discuss with you, such as nutrition, exercise, stress management, or physical therapy. A good doctor will refer you to the best source of expertise, which may include professionals who are not doctors.

Communicating with healthcare providers
Tips for your next visit

The following suggestions are intended for before and after general medical appointments, for new health issues and routine visits. There are three things that you can do to make the appointment go much better: *Do your homework, summarize your concerns, and follow-up.*

A list of questions to ask the doctor at the time of a new diagnosis is contained on page 75.

1   **Prepare for the appointment, and come with questions.** Doctors will appreciate working with you if you are prepared. You must be an active participant in your care.

2   **Don't expect your doctor to remember everything you talked about last time.** You'll need to keep track of that. It might be contained in their notes, but don't count on them reading the notes before the appointment. They might not have time to glance at them very long before they come in to see you. Doctors don't like to be short on time any more than you do.

3   **When you walk into a doctor's office, avoid acting or feeling like a victim, or that you have no control over what happens to you.** Most doctors are professional and respectful, but going in with the attitude that you are at their mercy will not help you. You truly are in control over what steps you take as you go forward. This is where preparation (in the form of designating an advocate, for example) will make health crises easier to navigate.

4 **Don't be afraid to ask your doctor to slow down and explain things**. When asking questions, it can be hard to understand the doctor's line of reasoning if you don't have a medical background. Be sure to slow your doctor down and have him or her back up and explain it in a different way. Doctors are used to using medical terminology and use it in their conversations unconsciously. Don't pretend to understand because you're afraid of looking stupid. Asking even the simplest question is smart!

5 **Get tests and blood work done ahead of time unless your doctor prefers you see him or her first**. Go with what the doctor recommends, and if their preference conflicts with yours, ask why so you understand their reasoning. They might be able to make it more convenient for you if they understand your needs.

6 **Answer the doctor's questions and be specific.** Tell them what you suspect about the problem, but don't tell your doctor that you know what the problem is. Give them time to gather information and assess you. You might think you know what the diagnosis will be, but they can determine a lot just by asking a few questions, listening, or feeling something. Give them a chance to practice medicine.

7 **Bring a copy of your list of medications, supplements, vitamins, and over-the-counter drugs**. It saves time during the appointment for you, the doctor, and their staff. Tell them everything (including herbs, vitamins, and supplements) that you are taking, because this is very important for your safety.

8 **On your medication list, include the name of the substance or medication, the exact dose you take, how often, and why you're on it**. Do not leave out any of this information. If you're not sure why you are on a certain medication, make sure you find out from the doctor who gave you that prescription.

9 **If anything has changed since the last time you saw the doctor, bring it up.** Try to limit the number of concerns to the most important ones and ask to see a nurse or make a follow-up appointment if there is limited time and you have a lot of questions.

10 **At the end of your appointment, very briefly summarize for the doctor what you heard him or her say, what you are expected to do, what the doctor will do, and when to follow-up.** Make sure you both understand each other, but don't make small talk. Let them move on to what they need to do.

11 **Get copies of anything you can't access on your own**. Even if you aren't in cancer treatment, stay on top of your medical records. You might feel like a professional patient, but it is in your best interest to know everything you can about your health.

12 **Stick to follow-ups with the doctor**. If your doctor tells you to come back in two weeks, do it. If they ask you to try something for a week or two, do it. Make the effort, and they will be more willing to work with you.

13 **Communicate about side effects and adverse effects after you start medication or treatment**. Your doctor needs feedback on how it is working for you.

14 **If you are given bad news:** A cancer diagnosis is rarely an immediately life-threatening event. If the doctor doesn't seem worried or in a hurry to get treatment scheduled, try not to panic. Your first impulse might be something like this, as one physician cancer survivor said of her own reaction: "Oh my God! I have cancer! You must cut it out NOW!" But if it were immediately life-threatening, your doctor would act immediately.

15 **Give feedback!** If you receive any kind of survey in the mail from a healthcare organization or doctor you have visited, it is essential that you fill it out, regardless of how good or bad the service was. This is the only way they will know whether they are meeting patients' needs. Whenever possible, mention names and dates. Give credit and thanks for good service, but don't hesitate to tell them if they did a poor job! Your long-term health depends on it, and many other patients are counting on it, too.

Athletes With Cancer

Athletes and other physically active people have a unique set of challenges with regards to cancer treatment. For example, they must consider the psychological, not just physical, impact of cancer on their ability to return to their sport.

Physicians are used to working with people who do not make such great demands on their bodies. Athletes can present a challenge to healthcare providers, as they may expect a higher level of physical and mental performance than the average patient. Athletes don't like when their performance is negatively impacted, and they usually want their energy restored quickly.

Finding support

A doctor may initially dismiss reports of fatigue or discomfort from an athlete, saying something like, "If it hurts when you run, don't run." But that is not an acceptable answer to a runner; running is an important part of their lifestyle and quality of life.

If your doctor is dismissive of your desire to train, find a doctor who understands what a return to full function means for you as an athlete.

How medical treatments affect athletes

Many athletes don't want to take medications for fear they will interfere with their performance. For example, if a doctor diagnoses an athlete with high blood pressure, many athletes will not want to take medications that lower their heart rate and cause exercise intolerance. The athlete needs a different medication, or a schedule for taking the medication, that minimizes the impact on their performance.

Weight gain and loss of muscle mass, reduced range of motion, neuropathy, or urinary or bowel incontinence are examples of cancer post-treatment effects that can be troubling to an athlete. Physical therapists and other rehabilitation professionals usually can provide considerable relief and guidance in minimizing debilitation and restoring function. You might be able to find support groups via social media for people with similar types of cancer. There are specific groups with information on how to manage the difficulties, what others have tried, what works well, what doesn't, and an idea of how long the effect might take to subside or disappear.

If you are facing chemotherapy that could cause damage to your heart, or if you need radiation or surgery that could reduce your function and range of motion, you must address this with your oncologist when discussing treatment options. Your future physical and emotional well-being depends on it. If you will require rehabilitation, discuss it and add it to the treatment plan.

If you need surgery, especially reconstructive surgery or other types that could affect your range of motion or muscles, joints, or bones involved in performing your sport, choose a surgeon who under-stands athletes' needs. Women athletes who have breast reconstruction surgery should seek out a surgeon who will work to preserve function in the upper body and avoid using donor sites for tissue reconstruction that might interfere with future performance.

Athletes can benefit from a coach's guidance to safely return to activity and performance after treat-ment. It takes patience and hard work but can yield good results. Know that it can take a year or more to return to previous activity levels, however, and you may see temporary or even permanent perfor-mance decline in some areas.

Emotional and social needs of athletes

Athletes' identities are frequently intertwined with their sport, social life, and lifestyle. Athletes often have strong social support networks within their sport. It's not unusual to see athletes' friends and training partners rally behind them during cancer treatment, doing support activities and even fundraisers. Despite all the support, it can be a very lonely time for an athlete with cancer.

In sports, athletes cheer each other on through tough times and help each other get to the finish line. For that reason, it's not unusual to hear other athletes telling the person with cancer, "You got this," "Fight," or "It's just another match." The person with cancer knows that it's not that simple and that there are no guarantees of a cure, however.

A good friend who understands how these sentiments are well-meaning yet inappropriate can help filter out some of the unwanted input by communicating your desires to other athletes you know. It's also a good time to find other interests to keep you mentally occupied so you avoid obsessing about what you're missing during treatment.

It's also important that your network understands you will not be able to work out at your previous level for some time during and after treatment. It's helpful to have a few friends who will train with you at your pace as you recover.

Patience and believing in yourself

Many athletes fear they will never return to their previous level of performance, but many factors determine how you will perform after treatment. Some athletes have been able to exceed their previous levels of performance. Remember that it took years to achieve your performance level. Athletes with cancer are not starting over from scratch, but they need to recover from the insult to their body that treatment has caused.

The most important thing is to allow your body to recover fully before you push yourself. You'll improve faster if you have fully recuperated than if you push your body when it still needs its resources for recovery.

Coming back after treatment

Be kind to yourself by not placing expectations or performance goals on yourself for some time after you return to training. General goals, such as progressing to a certain point, can be helpful, but try not to make them specific, and keep lower expectations. Relax, enjoy yourself, and try new things.

If the thought of not being able to do your sport, even for a short time, is so distressing that you feel unable to cope, speak with a counselor, preferably someone who understands athletes or has a sport psychology background. Heed the warnings and advice of your doctors and others who tell you to proceed with caution. By taking a break when you need to, you will save yourself a lot of time, frustration, and delays from illness or injury from trying to come back too soon. The "Goal-setting and Reframing" module on page A40 and at https://cancerharbors.com/table-of-contents-cancer-harbors/ helps in setting new goals.

84484255R00121

Made in the USA
Lexington, KY
23 March 2018